"This is it, finally! Most weight control books are one dimensional, focusing on the macronutrient, the exercise program, the magic bullet...but this is the all-in-one scientifically grounded manual to help readers lose the stubborn extra pounds and maintain a healthy weight for life!"

—*Alan Logan, bestselling author of* The Clear Skin Diet

"In *The Last 15: A Weight-Loss Breakthrough*, Dr. Shulman provides readers with an authoritative and, perhaps most importantly, motivating, no fail plan. She has written an empowering book that helps you to understand the intricacies of weight gain and offers accessible solutions so you can take control of your weight now!"

—*Jennifer Melo, of homemakers.com*

"A brilliant book. Dr. Joey gives us hope to deal with this critical health issue. This factual and informative book provides practical, easy steps to optimal health, along with a food plan that includes delicious, energy-packed recipes. This book will change your life."

—*Barbara Goodman, Editorial Director,* Canadian Health & Lifestyle.

"I wish this book was available when I was in the process of losing my excess weight. It would have armed me with the information necessary to stay the course and be part of the statistical minority that loses their weight and keeps it off."

—*Jamie Bussin, Publisher of* Tonic Magazine

"Anyone who takes an interest in their body and long term health should read *The Last 15*. Not only is it applicable, everyday advice, it's also easy to embrace Dr. Joey's recommendations. Many people struggle with the home stretch of weight loss; this is the perfect tool to help you get to the finish line!"

—*Tonya Rouse,* CityNews *Fitness Specialist*

the last 15

A WEIGHT-LOSS BREAKTHROUGH

the last 15

A WEIGHT-LOSS BREAKTHROUGH

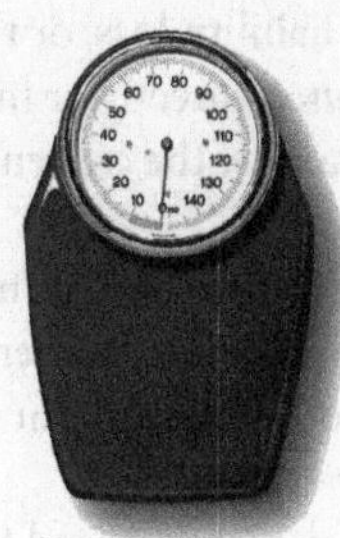

DR. JOEY SHULMAN

AUTHOR OF THE BESTSELLER *THE NATURAL MAKEOVER DIET*

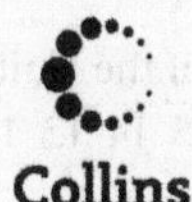

Collins

The Last 15

Published by Collins, an imprint of HarperCollins Publishers Ltd

Originally published by John Wiley & Sons Canada, Ltd.: 2008

First published by Collins in an EPub edition: 2013
This Collins trade paperback edition: 2014

HarperCollins Publishers Ltd
2 Bloor Street East, 20th Floor
Toronto, Ontario, Canada
M4W 1A8

www.harpercollins.ca

Library and Archives Canada Cataloguing in Publication
information is available upon request

ISBN 978-1-44342-793-7

Printed and bound in the United States of America
LSC 16 15 14 13 12 11 10

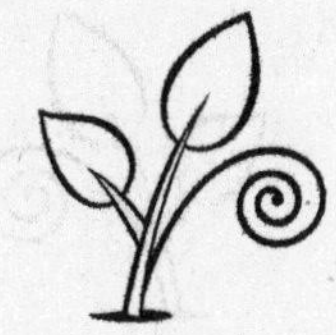

To my two heart songs Randy and Jonah, and
to my bubbi Elsie—the queen.

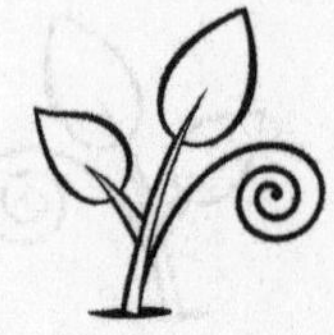

"Row, row, row your boat gently
down the stream
Merrily, merrily, merrily, merrily
Life is but a dream."

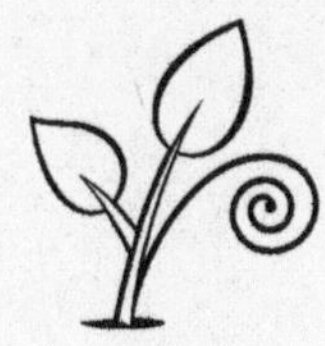

Contents

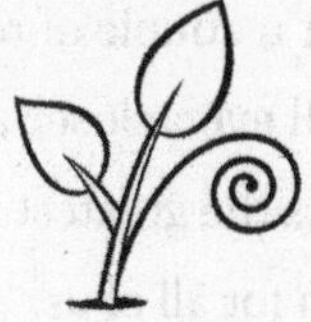

Acknowledgments

This book has been a joy to write from the first word to the very last. As I finish my third title—I stand back in a state of amazement and deep appreciation. I feel so blessed to be able to do something I love on a daily basis.

On my travels, I have had the privilege of meeting so many special people who have made positive health changes. From moms and dads to nurses and doctors—the stories I have heard of re-claiming health have served as great inspiration for this book. For those of you who take the nutritional information outlined in this book and make a difference in your health, the health of your families and communities—I say thank you and encourage you to spread the word on healthy living and eating.

This project has had many outstanding people behind it. To Ian Koo from Wiley for a beautiful cover design. A sincere thank you also goes to my editor Leah Fairbank for her diligent and thoughtful editing (and constant sunny disposition!). Thank you to Jennifer Smith for her continual support on this project and others.

One more big thank you to Helen Tansey for the cover shots—a dear friend and the best photographer I know.

To Justin, Sara, Myles and Codi—you continue to make us proud and we always look forward to being together.

To my group of girls who are there for everything...and I mean everything! I am blessed to have you all as lifetime friends.

To Danny, Laina, Sarah, Jamie, Matthew, Alex, Ben, Shane and Drew—I just needed to put your names down on paper because I love you all so much.

To my parents—oh what a couple of rollercoaster years it has been. If possible, it has made us all even closer and we are so happy for every moment we have together. As the greatest love story of all time, you both continue to be an inspiration for all of us.

On to my boys. To my husband and chef extraordinaire Randy—all readers will benefit from the delicious recipes you have created for *The Last 15*. As the "short-cut chef," you put the "easy" into healthy and delicious meals. In addition to making the best food on the planet...you are also the biggest "mentch" with the largest heart. To have you as my husband and best friend makes each day a great day.

To Jonah (bear)—the shiniest person I know. Thank you for filling our home with fantastic noise, chatter, laughter, love and pirate noises. We love you to the moon and beyond.

Randy and I would both like to pay tribute to our dear friend and producer Rick Pyman. His dedication to natural health, family and friends was extraordinarily unique and he will be forever missed. Cheers Rick.

Finally, to my bubbi Elsie—I am not so certain we will see the likes of someone like you again. So graceful, loving, strong and sweet. You are in my heart forever. A million will I's cookie, a million will I's.

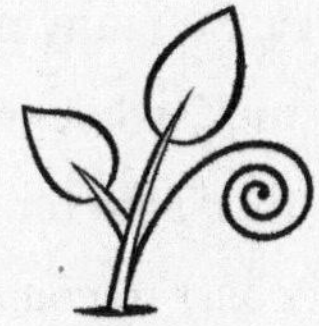

Introduction

"A man too busy to take care of his health is like a mechanic too busy to take care of his tools."

Spanish proverb

Are You Ready? Let's Do It This Time… for Good!

I have tried to lose weight…but I just can't seem to lose those last 15 pounds! This is a statement I have heard from hundreds of weight-loss seekers across North America. So many people have either lost weight only to gain it back and feel "stuck," while others want to lose but are confused about how to start. At the same time that all of these weight-loss attempts are occurring from coast to coast, the numbers of people now considered overweight or obese are growing at an alarming rate. In fact, statistics reveal that a startling 64.5 percent of American adults, or more than 120 million people, are overweight or obese. I don't blame people for feeling frustrated or intimated by the weight-loss world. With the bombardment of nutritional messages out there—points to count, low protein, low fat, a shake for breakfast, eating like the French—it is no wonder so many people are giving up and throwing up their hands in nutritional bewilderment.

After seeing the frustration of so many people on and off fad diets, I decided to set out not only to develop a nutritional program where anyone could succeed, but to also unveil the root causes of failed diets. In addition to identifying what was working, it was also important for the individual and North Americans to understand what was *not* working. I have often stated that the weight-loss industry is not a billion-dollar industry because it is working, but because it is not working! In fact, according to research done by Marketdata Enterprises in 1990, the annual revenue for the diet industry was over $30 billion dollars. This included diet centers, programs, books, magazines, trips to doctors and nutritionists, and exercise clubs with weight-loss programs. Consider some of the following weight-loss facts:

- The total retail market for weight-loss products and services in the United States was $84.7 billion in 2002. This market is expected to grow at an average annual rate of 13.2 percent through 2007 to $157.6 billion.

- The National Institutes of Health and other studies show that 98 percent of people who lose weight gain it back within five years. In other words, only 2 percent of all weight-loss seekers keep it off!
- 90 percent of those who lose weight gain back more weight than they lost.
- The Framingham study, published in The New England Journal of Medicine in 1991, found that the risk of dying from heart disease is 70 percent higher in those with fluctuating weights than in those whose weight remains stable, regardless of their initial weight, blood pressure, smoking habits, cholesterol level or level of physical activity.

With the end of the high-protein trend (Atkins) in 2003–2004, a slew of new weight-loss books popped up in the bookstores. From South Beach and the Sonoma Diet to the New York diet and the G.I. Diet—earnest weight-loss seekers had literally hundreds of titles to choose from. Although, for the most part, the information in these books was based on science and, as such, these books were excellent resources, the list of "what to do to lose" became too high and North Americans once again became confused on how to start. Programs and fitness centers also started to pop up on every corner outdoor mall. LA weight loss, Curves, the Dr. Bernstein Diet, Weight Watchers, Herbal Magic—which to choose? People would end up in my office asking me the same questions over and over again: Should I count points or restrict calories? Or is it better if I count fat grams or drink a shake for breakfast? The approaches were literally endless and were causing motivation to wane and frustrating weight-loss attempts that resulted in repeated failed attempts.

Thankfully, over the course of many years in the natural healthcare world as a clinician, writer and speaker, I have had the opportunity of helping hundreds of people reach their goal weight. I even had the unique opportunity to use these principles myself when I gained (and then lost) 70 pounds when pregnant with my son! The principles for weight loss and maintenance are what I call *The Last 15* or the "tipping point" to either optimal health or the slippery slope of weight gain and disease. Fortunately, once this pattern is identified and *The Last 15* food principles are implemented, reaching your goal weight and staying there becomes second nature and simple to maintain.

The Up-and-Down Pattern of Weight Loss

It is no secret that being overweight or obese is the most prevalent health concern of the 21st century. In addition to not looking and feeling your best, obesity-related diseases are at an all-time high and are the major killers affecting younger and younger generations.

Heart disease, cancer, hypertension, Type II diabetes and associated inflammatory conditions are all showing up in people in their 20s and 30s. In addition, being overweight has an enormous psychological effect that often goes unnoticed and undiagnosed. For example, in 2003, researchers set out to measure the quality of life of obese teenagers. Sadly enough, these youngsters rated their quality of life as equivalent to teenagers of the same age group undergoing cancer treatment such as chemotherapy. The good news is that re-setting your metabolic code and losing the weight dramatically reduces health and psychological risk factors.

More often than not, being overweight or obese is a mutli-faceted issue that is connected to both physical and psychological factors. The two key issues are:

1. Insufficient knowledge of nutrition and how it affects the hormones in the body.
2. The emotional component linked to *The Last 15*.

After years of witnessing hundreds of patients accomplish and sustain all their weight-loss goals, as well as interviewing thousands more, I now understand the core issues that lead to the inability to maintain a healthy weight for life. I have discovered an emotional and physical pattern as to why people get stuck in the weight-loss game. I will outline very specific nutritional principles that will prepare you for weight loss for life. In addition,

I feel it is imperative to examine the weight-loss world and identify why so many people get stuck on a metabolic roller coaster.

While *The Last 15* refers to a common phrase or statement often used, i.e., "I just can't lose that last ________pounds" (fill in the blank with how many pounds you have to lose), it also refers to the psychological breakthrough that is possible when you understand the core issues.

I have discovered in practice the four basic scenarios of dieting failure:

1. The person who achieves her goal weight for a short period of time but is not able to maintain it. This scenario is the most common and is often due to a fad diet that is overly restrictive or too hard to maintain—for example, weighing food, eliminating food groups such as carbohydrates, counting points or cutting calories to an extremely low level.
2. The "magic bullet" person. Like so many of us, this individual wants a pill for a quick-fix solution to weight. He has tried losing weight for short times, but gets frustrated and distracted easily. Stimulant metabolic boosters such as ephedrine or other supplements such as hoodia (a cactus-like plant said to decrease hunger) often appeal to this individual. These results are short-lived.
3. The "I have tried every diet in the world" person. This individual has literally gained and lost weight too many times to count. She is frustrated and has resigned herself to be overweight for life.
4. The 2 percent of the population who "get it" and take off the weight for good.

Do you identify with any of the above scenarios? If you are in category four and are among the 2 percent of people who have lost weight and kept it off for good—bravo! Take this book and give it to a neighbor, friend or colleague. However, if you are like most North Americans, who are still struggling with their weight, let's fix it, shall we?

A majority of people fall into categories one, two and three. Due to chronic dieting or faulty food choices they are out of balance hormonally and need to once again jump start their metabolism. By following the principles described in this book and implementing the 30-day food plan, "30 Days to Re-setting Your Metabolic Code," outlined in Chapter 4, you will quickly shed excess weight and improve your health both inside and out, mentally and physically.

What Is the Last 15?

When I decided to write *The Last 15*, I had mixed emotions. While in one sense I was excited and eager to share what I knew to be a weight-loss breakthrough with my readers, I also knew that there was great confusion in the weight-loss market that needed to be cleared up. With this large task in mind, I was determined to pen a book that would clear up past confusion that had arisen from recent fad diets once and for all. I did not want my readers to go on yet another program or fad diet. My motto for this book and weight loss is, "Let's do it ... and do it for good!"

The missing link with most weight-loss programs is the failure to deal with all three elements that are necessary to lose weight. *The Last 15* is truly a weight-loss breakthrough; it offers an approach to weight loss on all three critical levels.

1. **Physical**—30 days to re-set your metabolic code to lose weight, to increase your energy and experience an overall sense of well-being and enhanced beauty. (Bonus: improving your diet will improve the look and feel of your skin, hair, nails, etc).
2. **Emotional**—Hormonal balance through balanced meals improves your mood, makes it easier to avoid binge eating and decreases your cravings.
3. **Psychological**—Weight-loss success results in improved self-esteem and self- image, and provides constant motivation.

My research has uncovered that it is the combination of all three elements that creates long-lasting, sustainable weight loss. For example, if you cut out a specific macronutrient from your diet such as carbohydrates, you may lose weight temporarily; however, you will soon end up feeling deprived, fatigued and will experience intense sugar and starch cravings from being out of whack hormonally. Emotionally and psychologically this type of diet cannot create long-lasting effects. The reality is that this approach will lead to temporary weight loss and future weight gain. Frustrating isn't it? The same goes for extreme caloric restriction or other fad diets that do not deal with all the necessary components of weight loss. On closer inspection, it soon becomes quite obvious why a mere 2 percent of weight-loss seekers take it off and keep it off for good.

THE PERPETUAL MOTION OF WEIGHT LOSS

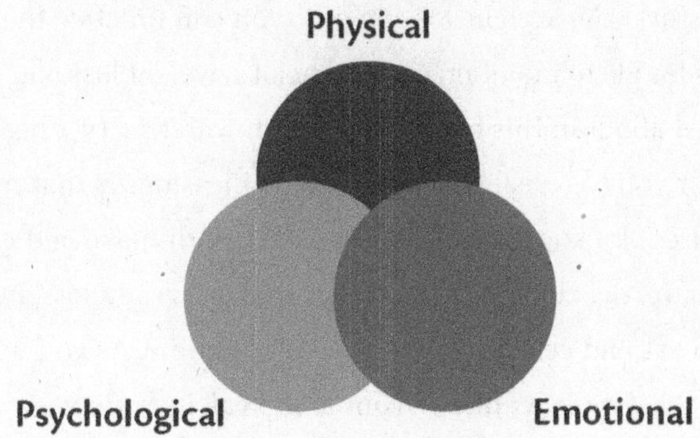

The three wheels above are what I refer to as the perpetual motion of weight loss. Each element is essential to long-term sustainable weight loss and each is co-dependant on the other. Think of this as a fly wheel. In other words, when one wheel has positive "pressure" put on it, e.g., through food changes, maintaining hormonal balance, etc., the other wheels start to spin, creating long-lasting and permanent changes. The combination of putting pressure on all three wheels spills over into one another and deeply imprints permanent weight-loss results. Without this multi-faceted approach, weight-loss results will likely be short-lived.

Of course, *The Last 15* is a book for diverse people, who have a variety of weight goals, not just losing 15 pounds. It is for the mom who wants to shed her baby weight and the 60-year-old who wants to lose his abdominal "tire." The principles in this book are researched, scientific and work for everyone. *The Last 15* refers to a "tipping point of health" that can determine the vitality, energy and quality of life you have in the future. Choosing to take care of those nagging few extra pounds—or ignoring them and letting them pile on—is one of the biggest determinants of your future health and wellness.

In this book, you will find that I refer to *The Last 15* as a set of principles, not a program. To me, a program suggests one that you can go "on and off." That is a recipe for failure and frustration. *The Last 15* is designed to create healthy habits that are quick, easy and sustainable for life.

While the first 30 days are designed to re-set your metabolic code and kick start your weight-loss engine, you can practice the remaining principles for life to maintain optimal health, weight loss and energy. The food talked about in this book is so mouth watering (yet healthy) it will be hard for you to resist. One of my many blessings is that my husband is the best cook I know. He has designed easy-to-make and grab-and-go meals that are delicious, healthy and geared for weight loss. In our house, we *love* to eat and celebrate with food all the time. As you will discover, the key is to enjoy every bite of your food in all its variety—with moderation and knowledge.

The first step is an initial 30-day food plan to re-set and re-boost your metabolic code. These 30 days are integral to success as they help to re-configure any damage done from previous weight-gain/weight-loss cycles. A specific map on how to get you to your own individual goal weight, depending on your height, weight, age and activity levels will help to ensure you take it off and keep it off for good. The next steps include core food principles to keep you on track, the exploration and connection between food and mood, how to shop for healthy grains and a look at the top foods to prevent the onset of disease.

Your Assignment

My goal is to make *you* part of that growing 2 percent who stops the weight-loss roller coaster. By applying the principles in this book, you will hit your goal weight, maintain it and enter a disease-prevention mode.

Here is what I am asking you to do. If you are reading this introduction, you are already motivated to lose weight and get healthy. Good for you! That is the first and most important step. My recommendation is to commit to reading this book in its entirety. Once you do, you will have the nutritional tools to set you up for life. You will be able to fall off the health wagon on occasion (as we all do!) and will then have the nutritional knowledge of how to get yourself back to the basics of health, both physically and mentally, and achieve your ideal body weight. Once you have this awareness and new information, you will be armed for life.

As soon as you sign on the dotted line, we, dear readers have a contract for health. I know you can do it! Are you ready? Let's do it this time... for good!

Wishing you best health,

Dr. Joey Shulman

Health Contract

I ____________________ (fill in your name) will reach and maintain my goal weight of ______________________(insert desired number). By signing this health contract I am committing to taking care of myself and becoming the healthiest me yet! I will read this book in its entirety and finally learn the nutritional tools that will keep me fit, energetic and at my ideal body weight for life! I am worth the effort.

Signature: ____

Date: ________________

part 1

The First 30 Days

1

The Tipping Point of Health: The Last 15

"Take care of your body with steadfast fidelity.
The soul must see through these eyes alone,
and if they are dim, the whole world is clouded."

Johann Wolfgang Von Goethe (1749–1832)
German poet, dramatist, novelist

Think back on your own personal health history. I am confident you can pinpoint a time in your life when the weight started to "creep up" on you. Whether it was an emotional trigger that got the number on the scale climbing, or the hectic pace of life that caused your health to take a back-burner position, one day you woke up and realized you did not feel like the vibrant, fit person you were meant to be.

The good news is that the body has an amazingly forgiving and restorative nature. Given the proper foods, nutrients and conditions, it responds positively in a very short time. I am continually amazed at the results I witness in my private practice. After people have abused their bodies for years—whether with smoking, stress, poor food choices, eating too much or lack of exercise—with the proper changes, they still bounce back to health and energetic living in one to two months' time!

I have found that the "tipping point" that decides whether you have a future of health, energy and disease-free living, or whether you end up gaining excess weight—triggering low energy, moodiness and a variety of associated disease (type 2 diabetes, heart disease, stroke and cancer)—all comes down to 15 pounds. Of course, *The Last 15* principles are applicable for people of all different sizes. It does not matter if you have five, 15 or 50 pounds or more to lose: the principles are scientific and, when applied properly, can work for anyone. The concept of the last 15 pounds means that it's a health crossroads.

In addition to outlining all the nutritional "need to know" that will get you to your goal weight (and keep you there), in this book I'll also examine why most weight-loss programs do not work. If only 2 percent of people are taking off weight and keeping it off for good, something is wrong. This is not your fault!

The current paradigm of dieting in North America is based on marginal and temporary progress that keeps you coming back for more. Think about the number of times you have been enticed by a weight-loss ad that promises that you'll take off 20 pounds by Christmas or drop two dress sizes in time for the beach. Weight loss is routinely marketed as a magic pill, limited-time offer that requires little investment of time and energy and often leaves your wallet feeling significantly lighter! It is also incredibly disheartening to lose 20 pounds on a "system" and then gain it all back. In addition, this constant up-and-down weight loss battle results in a sluggish metabolism on top of feelings of frustration, deprivation and despair.

Weight loss is also characterized as a lifestyle change. Most people equate that with sacrifice and constant discipline. As you will see in the delicious food options outlined throughout these pages, nothing could be further from the truth. Once you understand the principles outlined in *The Last 15*, you will be able to indulge in some of your favorite "goodies" without causing fluctuations in weight, mood and energy. Trust me, no one (certainly not me!) stays on the health wagon every day. Christmas, birthday parties, weddings and Thanksgiving come every year; indulging in "no-no" foods is bound to happen. By understanding the principles in *The Last 15*, you will have the working nutritional information that will equip you for life. In other words, when you do fall off the health wagon, you can climb back to ensure you do not gain back any weight lost.

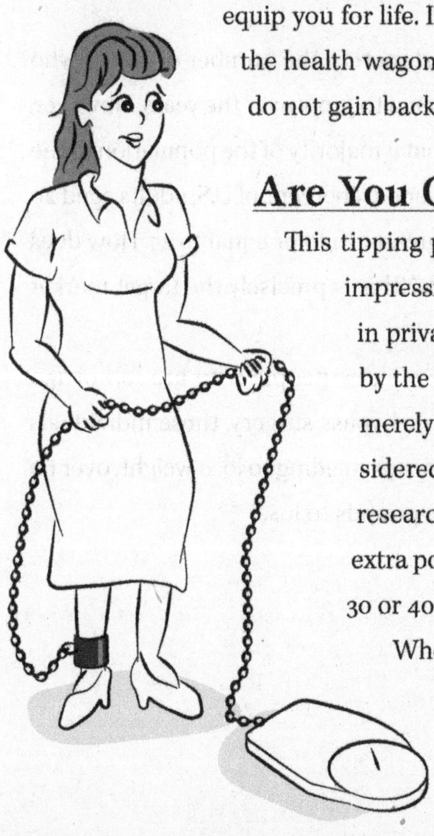

Are You Overweight?

This tipping point of *The Last 15* is not only my impression, and one that I have witnessed in private practice, it is also substantiated by the growing numbers of those who are merely somewhat overweight (but not considered obese). Remember, according to research, most people start with about 15 extra pounds. That eventually turns into 20, 30 or 40 pounds that need to come off.

When looking at the prevalence of people who are overweight and obese, the body mass index (BMI) is one of several measurements that are used to measure body fat. The equation is calculated as weight in kilograms divided by the square of the height in meters (kg/m2). Studies by the National Center for Health Statistics indicate that:

- bmi values below 18.5 are considered underweight.
- bmi values from 18.5 to 24.9 are healthy.
- Being overweight is defined as having a bmi between 25 and 29.9. A bmi of about 25 kg/m2 corresponds to about 10 percent over ideal body weight. People with BMIs in this range have an increased risk of heart and blood vessel disease.
- Obesity is defined as a bmi of 30 or greater (based on National Institute of Health guidelines)—about 30 pounds or more overweight. People with bmis of 30 or more are at higher risk of cardiovascular disease.
- Extreme obesity is defined as a bmi of 40 or greater.

As can be seen in Table 1.1, unfortunately, the number of adults who are overweight and obese has continued to grow over the years. However, the interesting story in this table is that a majority of the population in the United States is not obese. In fact, over 64.5 percent of U.S. adults aged 20 or older are overweight with a BMI greater than or equal to 25. How does this all start? With the last 15 pounds! This is precisely the target market of most weight-loss centers.

Even though media outlets often show people who are 100 or 150 pounds overweight who need gastric bypass surgery, these individuals are a minority. Of all the North Americans needing to lose weight, over 64 percent have only between 15 and 40 pounds to lose!

Increase in Prevalence of Overweight, Obesity and Severe Obesity Among U.S. Adults.

	Overweight (BMI > 25)	Obesity (BMI > 30)	Severe Obesity (BMI > 40ht
1999 to 2000	64.5	30.5.	4.7
1988 to 1994	56.0	23.0	2.9
1976 to 1980	46.0	14.4.	No Data

Source: CDC, National Center for Health Statistics, National Health and Nutrition Examination Survey. Health, United States, 2002. Flegal et. al. Journal of the American Medical Association 2002; 288:1723–7. NIH, National Heart, Lung, and Blood Institute, Clinical Guidelines on the Identification, Evaluation and Treatment of Overweight and Obesity in Adults, 1998.

Please note: In terms of assessing overall risk factors, the BMI calculation does have some limitations. It can overestimate body fat for athletes or those who have an extremely muscular build. It may also underestimate body fat in older persons and others who have lost muscle mass. For a detailed overall chart of the body mass index, please refer to the appendix.

Another diagnostic tool used to determine your amount of body fat and future risk factors is waist circumference. To measure your waist circumference, simply place a measuring tape snugly around your waist. This number is a good indicator of your abdominal fat, which is a predictor of risk for developing future diseases such as heart disease, insulin resistance and type 2 diabetes. The risk increases with a waist measurement of over 40 inches in men and over 35 inches in women. Please refer to the appendix to provide you with an idea of whether your BMI combined with your waist circumference increases your risk for diseases related to being overweight or obese.

What Is Health?

"Health is the greatest gift, contentment the greatest wealth, faithfulness the best relationship."

Buddha (568–488 B.C.)

Health is defined in a variety of ways:

- A healthy state, free from disease
- An absence of disease or injury, especially when accompanied by a general physical, mental and social wellbeing
- The overall condition of an organism, at some particular time, and in relation to a soundness of body or mind.

Our old, allopathic idea of health is disappearing. It's being replaced by a more up-to-date, integrative healthcare model, which now considers health from a broad wellness perspective. This model encompasses both medical care and the natural health world. Health is seen not just as freedom from disease, but as a more complete state of well-being: physical, mental and social.

Our current healthcare model incorporates a variety of approaches including medications, surgical intervention, diet, exercise and lifestyle and stress management. Even so, this model is experiencing a peculiar growth at present time. While giant leaps are being made on the science and applications of natural medicine, obesity-related illnesses are also at an all-time high. A study conducted in 2003 estimated that healthcare costs associated with obesity now rival those attributable to smoking. Researchers say obesity costs in the United States totaled up to $92.6 billion in 2002! On average, treating an obese person cost $1,244 more in 2002 than treating a healthy-weight person did.

While we hear these statistics constantly, there still exists an "it can't happen to me" attitude. When I gently explain to people that even carrying around a small amount of excess weight can increase risk factors for a variety of illnesses, I can see in their eyes that they think it will happen to others, not them. Now, I am not telling you this to scare you into losing weight. You must feel ready and want to make a change for yourself. I am confident that you are ready: you are reading this book. The good news is that by losing the weight, you will not only look your best on the outside—which will dramatically boost your confidence and energy levels—you will also enter a very powerful prevention mode that can prolong your life and reduce the risk of future disease.

Obesity-Related Diseases

Even though being 15, 20 or 30 pounds overweight may not seem significant, it is still enough to raise obesity-related disease risk factors, such as heart disease, hypertension, high cholesterol and stroke. This past year, I spent a week on a cardiac care floor. Even though I have worked for over a decade in the natural healthcare field, I was taken aback by the number of young patients in their 30s and 40s. The ward was filled with a generation of younger men who had suffered from heart attacks due to their weight, smoking and stress levels. In addition, all of them except for one were also diagnosed with type 2 diabetes.

Take a look at the most-prescribed medications to see which diseases are placing this enormous burden on the individual and on the healthcare system. Of the top 10 medications sold in 2005, six can be linked to being overweight. The most-prescribed medications for 2005 were the following:

Top 10 Medications in 2005

Drug Name	Total Prescriptions (x 1000)	Usage	Related to obesity or being overweight
Hydrocodone/ Acetaminophen	101,639	Used to reduce pain and fever	
Lipitor	63,219	Cholesterol-lowering medication	√
Amoxicillin	52,104	Antibacterial drug	
Lisinopril	47,829	Used to treat high blood pressure (hypertension) and congestive heart failure and to improve survival chances after a heart attack	√
Hydrochlorothiazide	42,757	Used to treat high blood pressure	√

continued

Atenolol	42,001	Used to treat high blood pressure. It also is used to prevent angina (chest pain) and treat heart attacks.	√
Zithromax	38,110	Antibiotic that fights bacteria	
Furosemide	34,782	A "water pill," used to reduce the swelling and fluid retention caused by various medical problems, including heart or liver disease	√
Alprazolam	34,230	Anti-anxiety drug	
Toprol-XL	33,598	Once-a-day beta-blocker for high blood pressure, angina pectoris over the long term, and heart failure	√

What about Genetics?

While it is true that everyone is put on this earth with a unique genetic makeup that can influence future health and disease, it is also true that environmental components such as diet, lifestyle, stress levels and smoking can also have enormous impact. Recognizing the immense effect of environmental factors, in 2005, researchers at the Harvard School of Public Health decided to test what they described as the "modifiable risk factors" for cancer—the changeable risk factors that people can control. The findings of this study were fantastic. The researchers concluded that more than one-third of the 7 million cancer deaths that happen every year worldwide were caused by nine avoidable and modifiable risk factors. In other words, 35 percent of all cancer deaths were attributable to nine behavioral and environmental risk factors. They are:

1. Overweight and obesity
2. Low fruit and vegetable intake
3. Physical inactivity
4. Smoking
5. Alcohol use
6. Unsafe sex

7. Urban air pollution
8. Indoor smoke
9. Contaminated injections from healthcare settings

Why do I call this research fantastic? Because the power lies within us to change our future health. Most people believe cancer is a disease "set in stone" and that outside influences are not that effective. However, we are now well aware that maintaining a healthy body weight, eating more fruits and vegetables, not smoking, exercising, drinking alcohol responsibly and practicing safe sex can decrease our cancer risks by 35 percent! This is indeed wonderful news.

Beyond cancer, nutritional and lifestyle changes can dramatically reduce risk factors for a variety of diseases, such as type 2 diabetes, heart disease, stroke and high cholesterol.

Why Start Now?

In one of my previous books on pediatric healthcare, I recorded a number of excuses parents had for why they could not feed their children healthy food options. I outlined the excuses early on in the book because I wanted to wipe the slate clean and have all parents begin from the same starting point.

In terms of weight loss, the word "excuses" implies that people are looking for an out so they do not have to start. I think excuses is too harsh a term in this case. However, I do believe most people who are frustrated with the weight-loss world (and are perhaps carrying some emotional baggage) have their own internal list of reasons why they "cannot lose weight." Here are some examples.

- "I am too tired to start."

  This is my favorite. This is precisely the reason you should start!

- "I don't have the money to start another program."

  You bought this book; you have to grocery shop anyway—there will be no more added expense, just focus.

- "All of my family is overweight; that's the way we are."

Not necessarily. While I agree that every body has a different shape and size, it is still integral to health that you maintain a healthy weight range. By doing so, you will dramatically reduce your risk factors for a multitude of disease processes, and you will boost your self-confidence.

- "I have tried every diet out there; they just don't work for me!"

  If you have tried every diet on the market, stop! Read this book in detail, sign the health contract in the introduction and take the time to understand the "what" and the "why" behind your eating. Until you do, permanent change is unlikely to happen.

- "This simply won't work for my family."

  It will. Improving your health by losing weight is a very important and honorable venture. Explain to your family that you need support on this. Also, as mentioned, you will not be eating plain tasteless tofu—your food choices will be delicious and bursting with flavor, taste and natural sweetness. If you have children, this is an even better reason to start on the right track. Children are "monkey see, monkey do" in terms of food choices and will eat whatever they find in the house—good or bad.

The Crossroads of Health

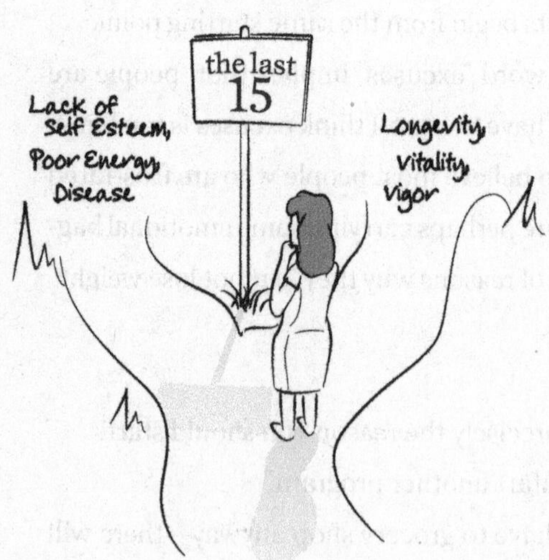

Remember, being overweight is not just about the number on a scale. It is a multi-faceted issue that involves emotions, hormones, food choices and is influenced by outside marketing. In this cartoon, we see someone standing at the crossroads of health. Let's call her Mary. Mary can take path

A or B, which will affect her future years of vigor, vitality and disease-free living. Like so many people, while standing at this crossroads, Mary is carrying an excess 15 pounds. Which path will she choose? Let's examine the possible two scenarios in order to highlight the crucial effect of those last 15.

Scenario 1: Ninety-Eight Percent of the Population

Mary is a 38-year-old, medium-framed woman and is the mother of a beautiful two-year-old boy. She is 5 feet 3 inches and currently weighs 150 pounds. At this height and weight, Mary's BMI is 26.6 (overweight). Mary gained 45 pounds while pregnant. Although she lost 30 pounds after the birth of her son, she was not able to shed those last 15 pounds. After trying two quick-fix solutions that backfired on her, Mary's weight has slowly crept up and is now the highest it has ever been. Mary is feeling depressed about her body, fatigued and unsure of what to do. She is extremely busy as a working mom and feels she does not have the time or energy to diet. Due to extreme frustration, Mary has succumbed to her current body weight and has decided to accept it.

Unfortunately, as Mary ages, her metabolism will slow even more. If nothing changes, her weight will continue to go up by one or two pounds a year. This will put Mary at risk for a variety of female-related disease processes: heart disease, hypertension (high blood pressure), type 2 diabetes, stroke, heart attack, cancer, gallstones and gallbladder disease, gout, osteoarthritis and sleep apnea.

Scenario 2: Two Percent of the Population

Now, let's assume Mary is 15 pounds overweight (as she is in scenario 1). However, fed up with the weight-loss world, Mary decides to get informed and acquire the tools to lose the weight for good. With a specific working knowledge of how to eat carbohydrates, proteins and fats combined with natural metabolic-boosting tips, Mary easily takes off the 15 pounds in five weeks and keeps it off for good. By doing so she has much more energy to chase after her son, is feeling much better about her body and has dramatically reduced her risks for a variety of obesity-related disease processes. Sound too good to be true? It is not—it can and will happen to you. You will be among the percentage of the population who takes it off and keeps it off for good!

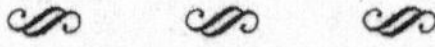

At the end of each chapter, I will share with you a personal story of a triumph of health. I will be introducing you to people I have watched lose weight for good by applying the principles in this book. These people are just like you and me, and now they understand how to balance health and maintain an optimal body weight, while enjoying delicious food.

Sharon

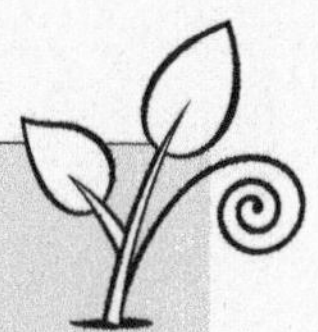

***Age:** 40*

***Height:** 5 feet 4 inches*

***Previous Weight:** 195 pounds*

***Current Weight:** 152 pounds*

***Total weight lost:** 43 pounds and still losing!*

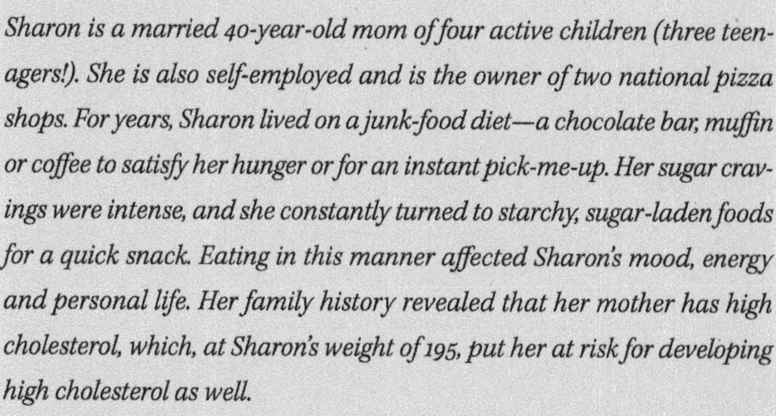

Sharon is a married 40-year-old mom of four active children (three teenagers!). She is also self-employed and is the owner of two national pizza shops. For years, Sharon lived on a junk-food diet—a chocolate bar, muffin or coffee to satisfy her hunger or for an instant pick-me-up. Her sugar cravings were intense, and she constantly turned to starchy, sugar-laden foods for a quick snack. Eating in this manner affected Sharon's mood, energy and personal life. Her family history revealed that her mother has high cholesterol, which, at Sharon's weight of 195, put her at risk for developing high cholesterol as well.

Sharon quickly lost 15 pounds in the first couple of months and continues to lose one to two pounds per week. Her energy has soared; she is less stressed and feels much better about her body. (As a hard-working mom and entrepreneur, she needs focus and energy throughout the day.) She no longer experiences "food hangovers" from eating refined high-glycemic index carbohydrates and nutrient-void food. Sharon's mood and self-esteem have changed so dramatically since she lost the weight, her story was told on a national Canadian news network. She is still losing weight but does not feel deprived in any way. She can enjoy delicious, hearty meals—with the occasional goodie. She keeps her "before" jeans (size 18) as a reminder of how far she has already come. Currently, Sharon is very proud to wear a size 10!

2

Getting Started

"Whether you think you can, or you can't—you are right."

Henry Ford (1863-1947)
Founder of the Ford Motor Company

Old habits die hard. This saying is especially true for food and dietary changes. On a very deep and intimate level, we are all connected to our food choices. Food signifies different things to different people. For some, it can help to soothe and comfort us when we have feelings of loneliness, despair or anger. For others, it may be used in excess for celebrations, in times of joy and as a reward for a hard day's work. Whatever the reasons, I am a firm believer that on some level, we are all emotional eaters.

To change any habit or make any significant lifestyle change you have to be in the correct mindset. A smoker cannot quit smoking unless he has made up his mind to do so. In order for effective change to occur, the motivation and desire for a different pattern of life has to be the underlying impetus. Weight loss and dietary changes are no exception. In fact, people often find dietary changes the hardest change to make and stick to. This is yet another reason why the current weight-loss industry is now a booming multi-billion dollar industry. The desire to lose weight is very personal and complex; you may have a variety of reasons for wanting to lose weight. You may want to fit into your little black dress at an upcoming reunion or, on a more serious note, you may have decided to get control of your health due to an illness or disease. The key is to know that once you acquire the correct information and set up an action plan, the results are easily attainable. Even better, once you complete the two stages outlined in this book, you will be hormonally balanced and ever-nagging food cravings and endless hunger will no longer plague you. The two stages described in this book will help you achieve permanent and long-lasting weight loss.

Stage 1: Thirty days—Re-setting Your Metabolic Code

Stage 2: The Rest of Your Life—Keeping It Off for Good!

Before delving into Stage 1 and Stage 2, let's first examine some core principles to creating effective, long-lasting weight-loss results.

Creating Change

When it comes to changing behavior, the first few weeks of change are the most critical. In the classic book *Psycho-Cybernetics*, the author, Dr. Maxwell Maltz, states that it takes 21 days to change a habit. Dr. Maltz, originally a plastic surgeon, first observed this phenomenon while working with amputees. Maltz noticed that it took amputees 21 days to stop feeling phantom sensations—pain or discomfort following amputation that feels as if it comes from the missing limb. Maltz took this 21-day theory and applied it to other areas of change and noticed it was true for them as well.

According to numerous experts, the brain produces neuroconnections and neuropathways. New pathways can be created but only if practiced for 21 days in a row. If followed correctly, by the fourth week of engaging in the new behavior, it is actually harder *not* to follow the new behavior than it is to resort back to your old ways. In other words, the key to successful behavioral changes is repetition, repetition, repetition!

Innately, human beings typically fall into a variety of patterns of behavior. After approximately 21 to 30 days of the same pattern, these patterns become habits and are engrained or "installed" deep within the pathways of the brain. This is why change is often so hard for us to achieve. Whether it is waking up at 6 a.m., exercising daily or reducing TV time, many people try for a week or so and then give up because they feel it is not working. The truth is, they have not held on to their new pattern of behavior long enough for effective change to occur. Keep in mind that changing habits, dietary or other, is a skill, and like all other skills, it needs both practice and technique.

In terms of food and dieting, the key to long-lasting change is to "uninstall" faulty food habits. The following chapters will teach you how to do this in a manner that lets you eat delicious food, keeps your hormones balanced and revs up your metabolism. However, as you will soon discover, you cannot remove one behavior without replacing it with another. The food choices will be healthy and delicious with lots of options that still leave room for indulgences here and there. Although you may be eager to get started on your road to fit, thin and optimal health at this very moment, I highly recommend first reading this chapter in detail. By doing so, you will understand the why behind some of the foods you have been selecting. After that, you can move on to Chapter 3, which explains the importance of metabolism in weight loss, and to Chapter 4, which details the 30-day approach to re-setting your metabolic code.

The first step to any change is awareness. I assure you, you are already at the awareness step because you have committed to reading this book. The next steps to achieving long-lasting change for permanent weight loss include:

1. Identify the results you want.
2. Develop an action plan that will achieve those results.
3. Examine the internal beliefs that are holding you back.

All of the principles outlined in *The Last 15* are based on these three steps. By properly implementing them, you will find that losing weight, keeping it off and feeling your very best will no longer feel like an effort. It will be a way of life that you will enjoy; you will soon forget your old ways and quickly discover that looking and feeling your best, both inside and out, is the ultimate pay off.

Identify the Results You Want

With any new venture, it is important to identify exactly what it is you want. Whether it is to boost your income by 50 percent, to lose 50 pounds or to buy a new home—you need to name it. While this may not seem as important when first starting out with weight loss, I assure you, it is. When I am taking a health history, one of my very first questions is, "What is your goal weight?" First, I want to know what pops into your mind as your ideal weight. Second, it is very useful to have your eye on the ball to keep your weight-loss goals focused and on track.

In order to get where you want to go, it is important to identify where you are now. In other words, we need to get you on a scale! Although this may be scary for some of you who have avoided and dreaded that number for so long, it is important to know your starting point. Whether you use a scale at the gym or a home scale, it is important to weigh yourself on the same scale each and every time to avoid inaccuracies.

Your weight is a grand total of your bones, fats, tissues and organ systems. While this number offers one piece of valuable information, at times, it can be misleading because muscle weighs more than fat. This is why there are a few other significant measurements to record. All you will need is a measuring tape and a pen. The additional measurements are called circumference measurements. You will find these numbers to be of great value in the next 30 to 90 days, when you lose a significant amount of weight and inches.

Measure Yourself

For greater accuracy, it is best to have a family member, friend or trainer help you take your measurements. If this information is too personal, you can take the measurements on your own.

Waist

To measure your waist circumference, place a tape measure around your bare abdomen. As a rough guide, your waist is the narrowest part of your trunk, or approximately 1 inch above your belly button. Be sure that the tape is snug, but does not compress the skin, and is parallel to the floor. Relax, exhale and measure.

Hips

Measure the hips around the fullest part of your buttocks with your heels together.

Thighs

Measure the upper thighs, just below where the buttocks merge into the back thigh.

Chest

Measure around the fullest part of chest.

Once you have taken your measurements, please record them below.

Current weight:______________

Circumference measurements:

Waist:____________________

Hips:_____________________

Thigh:____________________

Chest:____________________

Now that you have identified your starting point in pounds and inches, it is important to identify your goal weight. You can even record your goals for inches lost. Why is this important? Naming and writing down your goal, for any venture, adds strength to the goal. When you commit it to paper and visit your goal daily, it adds significant power to permanent change. Sound a little too out there for you? Trust me, it works.

My goal weight is:____________

My goal circumference is:

Waist:____________________

Hips:_____________________

Thigh:____________________

Chest:____________________

Note: Now that you have your circumference measurements, you can check your waist to hip ratio in the waist to hip ratio chart in the appendix. People tend to gain weight in specific areas. For example, fat can be located on the hips and buttocks or the abdominal area. A greater fat deposition in the abdominal area is referred to as an apple-shaped body type, whereas greater fat deposition in the hip region is referred to as a pear shape. Apple-shaped individuals, in particular, (women with a waist measurement of more than 35 inches or men with a waist measurement of more than 40 inches) are at a greater risk for health problems associated with being overweight or obese such as type 2 diabetes, high blood pressure and heart disease.

What Is a Healthy Weight Range for Me?

Ah! This is the million dollar question. When you visit the internet and investigate healthy weight ranges, most web sites offer the Metropolitan Life height and weight chart. This table was first created by the Metropolitan Life Insurance Company in 1943 and was slightly revised in 1979. Although the amounts in the Met Life charts are offered as an ideal body weight for a variety of frames depending on gender, they can reflect gross inaccuracies. The values are much too high for short people and much too low for those who are 5 feet 8 inches or taller. In addition, there is no modification for age or activity levels, e.g., the star athlete vs. the coach potato. Lastly, the weight of North Americans has grown significantly since 1979 and the chart does not encompass this new data. For interest sake only, the Met Life height and weight charts can be found in the appendix.

For a more accurate target weight, I would aim for a healthy body mass index (BMI) and a normal waist circumference. In addition, I think every person has a weight that they intuitively know they feel better at. For example, I was recently contacted by a 32-year-old man who wanted to lose weight. Although at such a young age he was already a millionaire from his highly successful landscaping company, his weight had spun out of control. At 6 feet 3 inches and 260 pounds, he was feeling sluggish, run-down and had already developed high blood pressure. When I asked him what his goal weight was, his response was that he felt his best at university when he was between 190 to 200 pounds. Perfect! He intuitively knew the weight he felt his best at. His goal weight would also land him at a healthy BMI of 24 and a normal waist circumference.

Another quick calculation to help determine your ideal body weight is:

- Women: 100 pounds of body weight for the first 5 feet of height, 5 pounds for each additional inch.

- Men: 106 pounds of body weight for the first 5 feet of height, 6 pounds for each additional inch.
- Add 10% for a large frame size, and subtract 10% for a small frame size.

Body Fat Percentage and Lean Body Mass

In addition to examining BMI and waist circumference, many healthcare professionals also record body fat percentage versus lean body mass. This is an important percentage to acquire, as two individuals can have the exact same height and weight, but may vary significantly in terms of their total body make-up.

Our bodies are made up of a number of tissues such as muscles, organs and fat. The body fat percentage of an individual is just that—the percentage of their weight which is made up of fat. The part of the body that is not fat is referred to as the "lean body mass." For example, an individual who weighs 160 pounds with a lean body mass of 110, has a 25 percent body fat (40 pounds of fat). Keep in mind that a certain amount of fat is necessary for health; it provides part of our natural insulation, stores energy and is used for hormone production. The problem arises when fat tips the scales in percentages and creates fatty build-up around our organs and arteries.

There are several methods to measure percentage of body fat, each different in reliability and cost. If you are interested in determining your percentage of body fat, the options are:

Skin-Fold Calipers (Pinch Test) This is a simple test but needs to be done by someone who is highly trained. It is not uncommon to find inaccuracies and wide fluctuations, depending on the person doing the test. It all depends on the skill of the individual measuring.

Bioelectrical Impedance (BIA) These are scales and hand-held devises that run low-level (and painless) electrical current through the body. You can often have this test done at your gym. However, while this measurement can be accurate, it also varies according to the specific device and how it is used. For optimal results, it is best to do this test in the morning and for the individual being tested to consume no alcohol for two days prior.

Hydrostatic Weighing This technique involves weighing under water (completely submerged, with all air blown out of the lungs). When done by a trained professional, this method is extremely accurate.

Navy Tape-Measure Method This is a formula used by the military based on several body measurements taken with a tape measure. It works and you can do it yourself, but it also depends upon your ability to accurately measure. All you will need is a tape measure and a scientific calculator. Please refer to the appendix for the calculation. (The calculation may be slightly confusing. If you would like to take the measurements and do the calculation online, there are several body fat calculators available that are free to use.)

Please refer to the charts below for healthy body fat percentages. Remember, do not confuse BMI or waist circumference with percentage of body fat. They are all different measurements. Do not panic if you become confused with all the different measurements (waist circumference, BMI, and percentage of body fat!) Once you have your initial circumference measurements and BMI as a baseline, you will be able to monitor your progress from many angles—pounds, inches and BMI changes. If you choose in the future to measure your percentage of body fat, the information in this book will assist you.

Percentage of Body Fat

Women

Age	Underfat	Healthy Range	Overweight	Obese
20–40 yrs	Under 21%	21–33%	33–39%	Over 39%
41–60 yrs	Under 23%	23–35%	35–40%	Over 40%
61–79 yrs	Under 24%	24–36%	36–42%	Over 42%

Men

Age	Underfat	Healthy Range	Overweight	Obese
20–40 yrs	Under 8%	8–19%	19–25%	Over 25%
41–60 yrs	Under 11%	11–22%	22–27%	Over 27%
61–79 yrs	Under 13%	13–25%	25–30%	Over 30%

Develop an Action Plan

In the following chapter, you will discover the steps to re-setting your metabolic code in 30 days. Why 30 days? In addition to taking 30 days to shake up your metabolism and get your metabolic engine running at high speed once again, on average, it takes an individual 21 to 30 days to imprint a new pattern of behavior before she will consider it second nature.

However, before we get started with the plan, there are powerful action steps you can take today that will create a supportive mindset for your coming weight loss. These additional steps are outlined below.

Create a Food Journal

Often times we tend to underestimate the amount of food we think we are eating. We gloss over some of the gory details of the two cookies we had with lunch, the can of pop with dinner and the two double-double coffees we had at breakfast. By doing so, we can underestimate our caloric intake by anywhere from 500 to 700 calories per day! Keep in mind, it takes a 3500 caloric deficit to lose one pound. That is 500 calories per day for one week. This can easily be achieved by tweaking here and there, but we need to know how many calories you are taking in to cut them down. As you read on, you will discover that the principles for weight loss in *The Last 15* focus on two necessary aspects 1) hormonal and 2) caloric balance. In the following chapters, you will also find nutritional tricks of the trade on how to save on calories without even noticing. There are several calorie counters on line that can help you get a general idea of how many calories you are eating daily. For starters, I highly recommend visiting www.caloriecounters.com.

In addition to ball parking how many calories you eat on a daily basis, food journaling also helps you to see the quantity and quality of the foods you are consuming. I recently was working with a man who said he really enjoyed drinking coffee. When I asked him to start recording his food intake in his food journal, it turned out he was drinking over 20 cups of coffee per day! We only began to see the major loop holes in his diet when he started recording in his food journal. In order to start, either invest in a small journal and start recording what you eat and drink daily, or refer to the end of the appendix for *The Last 15* food journal.

In order to get an accurate assessment of what you are eating, you need to keep your food journal for a minimum of three days. I can tell you, I find that the people who do the best with weight loss are also those who diligently keep a food journal in the first few weeks. It is important to accurately record everything—quantity, fluid intake, coffee, etc. You can simply pack your journal in your purse or scribble down what you have eaten at lunch or dinner and record it when you get home. If you choose to keep your food journal private from others, that is fine. Health is very personal and it is entirely up to you if you want to let people in on your weight-loss efforts. However, if you do decide to open up to others, I think you will be pleasantly surprised. Taking back control of your health is both admirable and of the utmost importance. Most people will outwardly applaud your efforts.

Visualize

Seeing is believing! When reading the biographies of the great leaders of our time, there is one common thread that is woven throughout their tales. These individuals saw the change they wanted to happen in the world before it ever took place. There are numerous stories of multi-millionaires or even billionaires, athletes, humanitarians and others whose accomplishments we admire: they all held a vision of what they wanted to achieve before it ever developed. It may feel a little awkward or even silly in the beginning, but it is all about training the mind to attract what you want and developing the behaviors to support that desire. If you do not feel the motivation to start visualizing, I have one word of advice—force yourself! Once you start losing weight and increasing your energy levels and mood, it will no longer feel like a chore to visualize your future.

In terms of weight loss, what you visualize is up to you. It can be an image of yourself in a tight black dress or looking svelte in a handsome business suit. You can also find a picture of when you were once at your ideal weight and paste it on your mirror or in a private area that you can look at daily. Visualizing an image of being trim and healthy will help to deepen the imprinting that is going to take place over the next 30 days. However, you have to do it every day. Every opportunity you have, whether driving to work, in your morning shower or in the gym working out, keep seeing the image that represents a fit and healthy you.

Is Something Holding You Back?

The final stage of permanent change is to examine if your internal belief system is holding you back. In other words, is there internal dialogue that is making it impossible for you to commit to this new program? If so, it is time for a change. This is one of the reasons why the principles outlined in this book are a weight-loss breakthrough. Gaining or losing 15 pounds will either tip you towards health and wellness or towards a state of future illness, both physically and mentally. In order to make sure you are choosing to go in the right direction, you need a dual approach. In addition to changing your eating habits and switching to fresh, whole food that will keep you satiated, free of cravings and will work to help the pounds melt away, you will also be implementing scientific techniques that imprint these on your mind as permanent changes. This is why I highly recommend exploring the emotional relationship you have with food.

Do you eat when you are sad? Bored? Depressed? Our food choices have a dramatic effect on our hormones, the body's most powerful chemical messengers. Not only will eating the wrong foods trigger hormonal fluctuations leading to weight gain, your mood will also be affected. I am sure you have had the experience of feeling sad, cranky or irritable after a food binge. The key to lifelong weight management success is not only to understand what, when and how much food to eat (more on this in the coming chapters), but also to clear away old food beliefs and make way for a new, healthy relationship with eating.

I recently began working with a beautiful woman who had over 100 pounds to lose. She was dynamic, energetic, smart and worked in the beauty industry. Although we did all the correct things—started a food journal, created meal plans, visualized and had one-on-one coaching sessions, etc.—she was not able to change her dietary intake for longer than a week or so. After a few weeks, I soon discovered that there were significant internal beliefs that were holding her back. She opened up to me and described food as her "best friend...worst enemy." In hard times, food was what comforted her and got her through turbulent feelings and experiences. Even so, she described the way she currently felt as embarrassed and even "dirty."

I can tell you, to meet this young woman was to instantly fall in love with her bubbly nature and generous spirit. Where did all these negative emotions stem from? As we continued our one-on-one coaching, she revealed to me that her father had left her mother years ago because her mother had gained a considerable amount of weight. I suggested that perhaps she felt that losing the weight would hurt her mother. She agreed and felt that there were deeply ingrained internal beliefs about being thin and feeling good that were holding her back. On an emotional level she did not feel worthy enough to lose the weight and was fulfilling a false belief system that her father had ingrained in the family unit. Until we dealt with these internal beliefs on a deeper level, permanent nutritional changes were far less likely to stick.

So how do you change your internal belief system that may be holding you back? This is a process that you can do by examining your thoughts. Sit down in a quiet room and write out the answers to these questions:

I eat the most when I am... (hungry, sad, happy, alone, unfocused):

____

____

____

____

I am currently overweight because of... (emotions, experiences, schedule, poor eating habits, etc.):

____

____

____

____

If I were to name one issue that is holding me back, it would be:

____

____

____

____

In the future, when you do fall off the health wagon and eat all the wrong foods—fast food, cakes, cookies—ask yourself why. Keep in mind there is a difference between overeating occasionally at a dinner party or a wedding and indulging in repetitive food binges. Once you can be honest and open about the why behind your emotional eating pattern, you can change it.

I also recommend watching your internal dialogue. Constantly telling yourself you are fat or unworthy of being your ideal weight is detrimental to your success. Replace these thoughts with a positive mindset such as, "I am on my way to my goal weight," or "I am a beautiful, fit woman." You can say a positive affirmation statement over and over again to help with the imprinting of health changes you want to install over the next 30 days. If you are uncomfortable with your size and have decided to finally reduce it by following the principles outlined in *The Last 15*, bravo! But do it in a positive manner that keeps the weight off for good. If you do fall off the health wagon, do not crash the cart completely—just climb back on and continue on your road to success. Trust me, food guilt gets you nowhere fast.

If this feels like an impossible venture or too hard a journey to embark on by yourself, you can also lean on a trusted friend or counselor to help you get to the bottom of these issues.

There Is No Plan B!

I recently overheard someone ask a client of mine, "What will you do if you do not reach your weight-loss goal?" His answer was, "There is no plan B—this will happen." Perfect. This sort of determination, motivation and dedication will allow this gentleman to achieve any and all of the goals he sets for himself in the future. Remember, as William Shakespeare so eloquently said, "To thine own self be true." These words encompass one of the most important life lessons that will help to pave a path towards happiness and wellness. Being healthy, feeling vibrant, energetic and focused is your birthright. If you are not at that point now, know that pursuing health is a very honorable, though sometimes difficult, venture—especially at first.

You may find that on your weight-loss journey you encounter those who poke fun at your attempts or even encourage you to eat all of the wrong foods! Try to keep a mental distance from any negative comments that may throw you off course. Keep in mind your end goal by reviewing your goals, visualizing and implementing the food changes outlined in the following chapters. You will soon have people asking you on a daily basis, "How did you do it?" Remember, there is no plan B!

Harvey

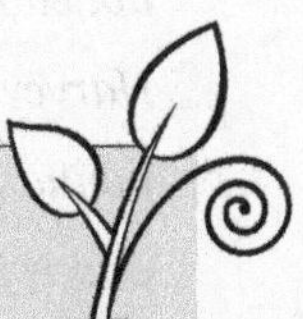

Age: 55

Height: 5 feet 7 inches

Previous Weight: 220 pounds

Current Weight: 180 pounds

Total weight lost: 40 pounds!

Harvey is a 55-year-old journalist who has struggled in the past with the ups and downs of weight loss. He had lost over 40 pounds in the past with high-protein and caloric restriction diets but was never able to keep the weight off for good. Harvey also identified himself as an emotional eater and attended a support group that helped address his emotional ties to overeating. He experienced mild to moderate depression and was on anti-depressant medications.

When I first met Harvey, his honest and kind nature and openness to change was instantly apparent. At 5 feet 7 inches and 220 pounds, his BMI was 35.2 (obese), which put him at risk for heart disease, high blood pressure and certain types of cancers. After submitting his meal plan to me, it was apparent that Harvey was eating far too many of the wrong types of calories. From high-glycemic index flours to an abundant amount of saturated fat, Harvey's nutritional intake needed a significant overhaul. In addition, he was completely dehydrated (making weight loss much harder) as he was drinking 20 cups of coffee per day. His daily diet consisted of sugary muffins, refined flours, fast foods and huge portion sizes that he often consumed at night. I sat down to figure out his daily food intake:

Calories = 3000

Grams of protein = 110

Grams of carbohydrates = 440

Grams of fat = 100 grams with 21 grams of saturated fat!

After only one month of nutritional changes that included cutting his coffee back to three cups per day, boosting his water and green tea intake, not eating past 7 p.m. and replacing all refined flours with whole grains, Harvey shed 15 pounds. As I write this passage, Harvey has lost over 40 pounds and has kept it off. He does not experience sweet cravings at night and is far less prone to emotional eating.

Are you ready to start? Let's move one step closer to embarking on the 30 days to re-setting your metabolic code.

3

Metabolism Matters!

"The groundwork of all happiness is health."

Leigh Hunt (1784-1859)
British poet, essayist

When discussing weight loss and dieting, the term metabolism often gets thrown around. If you have difficulty losing weight, it is thought that you are one of the unlucky ones who have a "slow" metabolism dooming you to a future of continued weight gain and weight-loss struggles. If you have a "fast" metabolism, you may be among one of those lucky few who can eat anything and everything they wish, never gaining a pound.

The question that researchers and doctors have been investigating for years is whether metabolism can be altered through various lifestyle and dietary changes. Science demonstrates with great strength that the answer to this question is a resounding yes!

Too Much of a Good Thing?

Increasing your metabolism can be tricky business. You must strike a fine balance between caloric intake, proper food choices and exercise. If you go too extreme on any of of these, your metabolism can respond as though you are in a pre-historic time of starvation: it will go into a "safety mode" of storing fat and calories. In other words, your metabolism will do exactly the opposite of what you want it to do. Balance is key, and this chapter will show you just how to do it right.

In this chapter, we will explore everything you need to know about metabolism. Then, in Chapter 4, I will explain the steps to re-setting your metabolic code in just 30 days. Why 30 days? You now know it takes a minimum of 21 days of continual and constant change to make permanent changes in the brain's pathways. As we saw in Chapter 2, our food choices consist of much more than what we eat on a daily basis. We have a deep emotional and physical link to food that requires changes on many levels. Plus, when starting to lose weight, the first 30 days set the stage. In order to properly rev up your metabolic engine and start losing weight effectively and on a continual basis, it is critical to be as strict as possible for the first 30 days.

How Much, How Fast?

The question I am always asked by clients is: how much weight will I lose per week? And my answer always is: it depends. At minimum, you should be losing two pounds per week in the next 30 days. If you are losing two pounds per week, you are on the right track. However, more often than not, in the first month of weight loss, you will lose more than that (partially due to water loss). On average, I have found that my clients lose three to four pounds per week or more in the first month. I recently saw a very popular program that advertises that you can lose eight to 10 pounds per week. This is not healthy for your body, mind or for keeping it off in the future. Severe caloric restriction or diets that are high in protein are famous for working only in the short term. I have met many hard core "Atkins" or "Bernstein" dieters, who report feeling extremely low on energy, moody and constipated from lack of fiber in their diet. You do not need to suffer these side-effects of weight loss. I assure you: you can lose weight and feel great at the same time. As you saw from the Framingham study quoted in Chapter 1, it is far worse for your health to lose and regain weight repeatedly. Losing two pounds per week, or slightly more depending on your individual make-up, is within a healthy range. If you are not losing at a rate of two pounds or more per week, refer to Chapter 5 to find out why and learn some tips that will help.

Do Not Weigh Yourself Daily!

I cannot stress this enough. This will only lead to frustration and a burst in your weight-loss bubble. Staying motivated and seeing results is just as important as eating the right foods. Weight-loss changes do not take place overnight. Weigh yourself on the same scale once per week in the morning. Record your weight from week to week to monitor your progress.

What Is Metabolism?

The majority of people feel their metabolic rate is fixed and cannot be changed. While some aspects that determine your metabolic rate are fixed (your age and gender, for example), as you will soon discover, there are many things you can control that influence your metabolism. This is why we see those who follow the principles outlined in *The Last 15* and re-set their metabolic code lose 15, 50 and even 100 pounds for life. The key is to maximize the aspect of your metabolism that is flexible; this ensures you triumph over the weight-loss battle once and for all.

Aspects that can influence the rate at which your metabolism functions include:

- **Age** Your metabolism actually slows about 5% per decade.
- **Gender** Men's bodies naturally contain more muscles. Muscle is far more metabolically active in comparison to fat. Thus, it is indeed harder for women to lose weight vs. men.
- **Genetic differences** Two individuals can have the same weight and fat content but have different body types, which result in different metabolic rates.
- **Hormones** Hormones control many of the body's main chemical processes and therefore can influence metabolism.
- **Lifestyle** A sedentary lifestyle can dramatically slow metabolism.
- **Underactive thyroid** The thyroid gland is a small organ at the base of your neck. One of the thyroid's roles is to produce hormones that influence your metabolism. When these hormones are in short supply, you have a condition called hypothyroidism. In addition to an inability to lose weight, fatigue, depression, dry skin, coarse hair and an intolerance to cold, there are other symptoms that can accompany hypothryoidism. Although, there can be several reasons why some indiviudals' metabolism is slower than others', thyroid problems are not usually to blame. A simple blood test by your medical doctor can help to detect if your thryoid is an underlying issue.
- **Skipping meals**
- **Chronic dieting**
- **A diet high in sugars and high glycemic-index carbohydrates**
- **Dehydration** Lack of water can slow metabolism.

- **Stress** When your body is stressed or in a chronic low-grade stage of emergency called "fight or flight response," you will over-secrete a stress hormone called cortisol. Cortisol secretion stimulates fat cells in the abdomen to increase in size and encourages fat storage. Excess abdominal weight is a risk factor for diabetes, heart disease and cancer.

Your metabolism can be likened to that of an engine. It uses food as the fuel to run your body. Similar to an engine, your metabolism can be sped up or slowed down. There are three aspects that make up your total metabolic engine.

1. **Basal metabolism** This accounts for approximately 60 to 65 percent of your metabolic engine. In a nutshell your basal metabolism amounts to the calories burned daily to keep you alive and provide basic energy for life support. In other words, if you were to lie around in bed all day long, you would still need these calories to provide basic bodily functions. An individual with more lean body mass will have a higher basal metabolic rate (BMR) than a person with a higher body fat percentage, even if he weighs exactly the same amount. Why? Because his body needs more energy to support and sustain his muscles.
2. **Physical activity** Approximately 25% of calories burned go to movement and physical activity. Muscle is more metabolically active than fat, burning 30 to 50 more calories than fat per pound per day.
3. **Thermic effect of food** About 10 percent of calories are spent processing the food you eat. For example, if you eat 2000 calories a day, you should be burning 200 calories a day through the process of digestion.

As you can see, the elastic part of your metabolism comes down to activity and food. These begin the tipping point outlined in *The Last 15*.

In addition, by focusing on these flexible aspects through proper food choices and exercising, your BMR can be increased, resulting in more calories burned everyday.

THREE ELEMENTS OF METABOLISMN

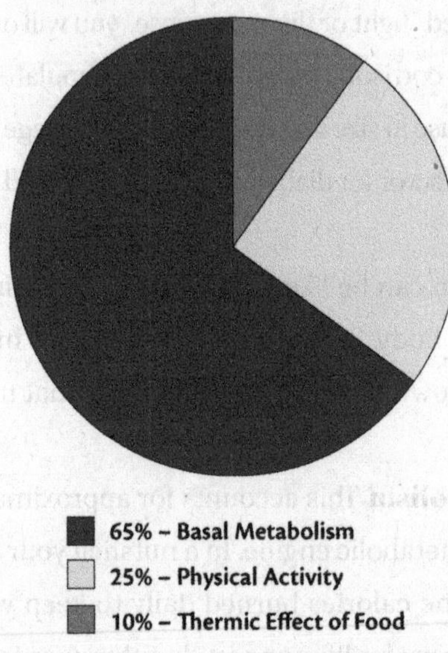

When understood and used correctly, these principles will keep you fit and trim for life. Remember, we will all fall off the health wagon from time to time. This concept can be referred to as the 80–20 rule of eating. In other words, by eating delicious and healthy foods 80 percent of the time and indulging in the foods we know are bad for us 20 percent of the time, we will still reach our health and weight-loss goals. My goal is to teach you the principles for weight loss and optimal health so that when you do over-indulge at a wedding, on a weekend or at a Super Bowl party, you know how to get back to your good eating habits.

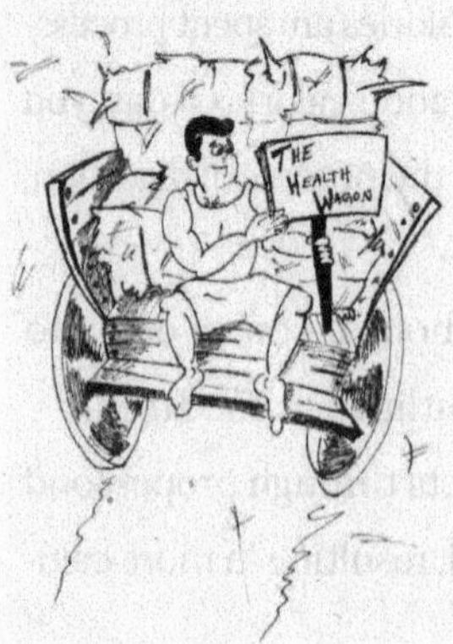

I have seen many people avoid the middle-aged spread simply by applying the principles in this book. The key is to know the steps you have to take to crank up the internal flame of your metabolism for good. This understanding is the greatest health tool you will ever have.

Calories vs. Hormones

Calories

When revving up your metabolic engine, there is a fine balance you need to strike between eating enough (and not too few) calories and maintaining hormonal balance. While some may think weight loss is a simple calories-in and calories-out equation, on closer inspection, it is more complex than that. By reviewing many years of weight-loss research, it is evident that both hormones and caloric balance are equally important and go hand in hand for permanent weight-loss success.

There are several popular diets that recommend going extremely low on calories and fat. On closer inspection, it is clear that science does not support these diets. When the body falls too low in terms of calorie intake, it enters *starvation adaptation mode*. In other words, in order to protect you, your metabolism slows down to conserve energy. Fat stores are saved due to what your body perceives as an emergency situation. Your body uses lean tissue or muscle to provide the calories it needs to function. This leads to a loss of muscle mass, which in turn lowers metabolic rate and slows weight loss. In other words, the body thinks it is starving. You did not know your metabolism could think, did you? Well, it is more like internal programming than a thought process. Your metabolism is programmed to keep you alive by burning fuel that comes in in the form of food. If your metabolism is sent a message that food is in short supply, it will take every opportunity to keep you healthy and safe by storing calories. Of course, this is an excellent adaptation mode if you are going through a time of famine, but not that great if you are trying to lose weight!

This is why I see so many desperate men and women eating very low-calorie diets and skipping meals, yet not losing a pound. Frustrating, isn't it? Instead of over-eating, these people are not consuming enough calories and are likely not eating as frequently as they should. In addition, going on a very low-calorie diet is not realistic, nor can it be maintained in the long term. Therefore, if you do lose weight (which you eventually will) on a very low calorie diet, you will quickly gain it back when you once again start to eat normal amounts of food. To top it off, very low-calorie diets can instill feelings of deprivation, which result in food binges and poor food choices.

In the first 30 days of my program, you will need to eat quite often. If you are following the steps properly, you should not be hungry at all, and your previous cravings for sweet and salty foods, which often occur around 3 p.m. and late at night, will subside within seven to 10 days.

During the first 30 days, your caloric range will be approximately 1300 to 1500 calories daily. Because the food you consume during the 30 days will be dense in nutrients and light in calories, you will find you are able to consume a lot of food. In addition, eating the proper amount of proteins, fiber and fat will keep you feeling more satisfied, your energy up and your weight down.

Hormones

Hormones are the body's most powerful chemical messangers. They can be likened to a very intricate phone system that connects thousands or even millions of messages with their intended recipients. You can imagine how chaotic it would become if this system was only partially working, or if messages were being sent to the wrong place. Because hormones are one of the body's master messengers that all intertwine with each other, hormonal health is a critical factor in weight loss and disease prevention.

As you will learn, eating too many of the wrong foods such as high-glycemic index refined flours and sugars will cause havoc to your hormonal systems and make weight loss nearly impossible. For example, eating too many high-glycemic index carbohydrates in the form of white bread, pasta, potatoes and sugary cereals will over-stimulate the hormone insulin, a fat-storage hormone.

On the flipside, recent popular diets use hormones to their advantage for weight loss, but with a disregard for the overall effect on health. For example, high-protien diets trigger the release of a hormone called glucagon, the opposite of insulin. Glucagon breaks down fat, and in turn pounds are lost. However, as you will discover, the body does *not* want to run on protein in the long term. While such diets make you lose weight initially, diets too high in protein are not sustainable or healthy over time; in addition to eventually gaining the weight back, individuals on high-protein diets report feeling lethargic, moody and constipated, and in extreme situations, they can develop inflammation that can be deterimental for heart health.

To add fuel to the hormonal fire, stress levels can also upset hormonal balance, causing an increase of the hormones cortisol and adrenaline. Fat cells around the belly love to attract cortisol, creating a situation of fat storage and increased risk factors for disease. As you can well see, there is no way around it—hormones need to be balanced for weight success. While the majority of the nutritional changes will focus on the interplay between insulin and glucagon, other examples of hormones involved in the "weight-loss game" include:

Growth hormone Released from the pituitary gland in the brain, growth hormone secretion increases with aerobic exercise. During exercise, growth hormone decreases the use of glucose and increases the use of body fat.

Endorphins Endorphins are your "feel good" hormones. They too are secreted by the pituitary gland. Endorphins help to boost energy, e.g., they are what give you "runners' high," suppress appetite, and reduce tension and anxiety. In addition, the more you exercise, the more sensitive you become to endorphin release, making longer workouts easier.

Testosterone Testosterone is a hormone produced by the ovaries in females and by the testes in males. Testosterone plays a role in increasing basal metabolic rate and decreasing body fat. It also affects the libido. Women have approximately one-tenth of the testosterone of men; these levels decline as they approach menopause. Men's testosterone starts to decline at approximately age 40 and up. Blood levels of testosterone can increase with exercise in men.

Estrogen Similar to testosterone, estrogen can boost libido, basal metabolic rate and mood. Estrogen decreases with age but can be increased by a certain degree with exercise in women.

Thryoid hormones Thyroid hormones such as T4 (thyroxine) raise the metabolic rate in the body and and help you to burn more calories. Stress, lack of exercise and genetics can effect thyroid function.

Fortunately, *The Last 15* strikes the perfect balance between caloric and hormonal intake, thereby sparking the metabolic engine for life. It maximizes the flexible part of your metabolism, contributing to your permanent weight-loss success. In addition to feeling fit and lean, you will also be eating a delicious diet that helps to prevent disease and supports aging optimally and gracefully. What could be better?

Now that you understand the importance of metabolism, calories and hormones in achieving your weight-loss goals, you are ready to start the 30 days to re-setting your metabolic code.

Kelly

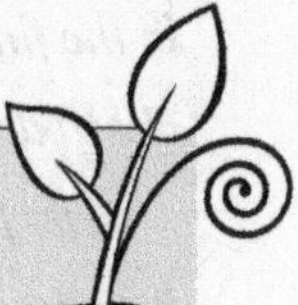

Upon first meeting Kelly, like so many other people, she told me of her previous weight-loss attempts. In her words, "If there was a book I read it; if there was a program I tried it!" Sick and tired of the ups and downs of weight loss, Kelly was ready to get healthy and take off the excess weight for good.

Kelly was instantly likeable; I was impressed by her intelligence, motivation and eagerness to change her health. With her slightly Type A personality and joie di vivre, *I knew this girl was a winner. Kelly also had a special wish that was the perfect goal for us to focus on to hit her goal weight: she was to be married in a year and in six months she wanted to buy her dress several sizes smaller than her dress size at our first meeting. Her goal was to lose a minimum of 30 pounds for the big day.*

Kelly explained that she first gained weight due to poor food choices and lack of exercise. Her job in the financial service industry involved a lot of travel, which meant she was on the road and staying in hotels a good part of the time. Because of this, she was grabbing refined and quick food choices such as cookies, bagels and muffins without even thinking. These sugary and refined carbohydrates were making her blood sugar soar, making her feel tired and making her gain weight. Kelly was also eating a lot of meals with trans fats, hidden calories and food additives such as pre-packaged dinners and frozen entrees. In addition, due to her lack of exercise and faulty diet, Kelly's bowels were incredibly sluggish; she only had a bowel movement once every three to five days. Her body mass index (BMI) was quite high at 32.3, increasing her risk for cardiovascular disease, stroke and cancer.

After our initial meeting, Kelly immediately started making nutritional and lifestyle changes. Accustomed to graphs, pie charts and time lines in the financial world, Kelly was eager to create a weight-loss graph that charted the pounds and inches she lost each week.

Her first major change was to eliminate refined flours and sugars from her diet, substituting whole grains, vegetables and fruits. Due to her hormonal fluctuations and over-secretion of insulin from chronic weight-loss attempts, it was also important for Kelly to introduce a lean protein such as turkey, chicken, fish, soy and eggs at each and every meal or snack. Kelly also became educated on the right types of fats to eat for weight loss, skin health and general wellness. On many occasions, she commented on how pleasantly surprised she was that eating healthy was so delicious and satiating!

Initially, Kelly's weight-loss journey got off to a bumpy start, while her digestion and elimination were being corrected and normalized with high-fiber foods and probiotics (good bacterial flora) such as acidophilus and bifidus. Kelly was also taking a multi-vitamin and fish oil supplements to optimize health, boost energy and aid in digestion. With determination and great will, Kelly cleaned up her diet successfully, balanced herself hormonally and rid herself of constant cravings. She also increased her energy dramatically and feels her skin now has a much healthier glow. I am happy to report that as I write this passage, Kelly is down over 30 pounds and is now the proud owner of a beautiful wedding dress, exactly the size she was hoping for.

4

30 Days to Re-Setting Your Metabolic Code

"Health is the condition of wisdom, and the sign is cheerfulness—an open and noble temper."

Ralph Waldo Emerson (1803-1882)
American poet and essayist

Now that you understand the flexibility of your metabolic engine, all you need are the correct steps to start implementing changes. The next 30 days are the most important in setting the stage for you to lose weight permanently and your health to flourish. Once the 30 days are finished, you will find more leeway in your dietary intake, and most important, you will have the tools and information to keep your metabolic engine revved for life. In this chapter and in chapter 5, I will give detailed meal plans, shopping lists and address commonly asked questions that you may have in the first 30 days.

Keeping in mind that it takes a minimum of 21 days to form a habit, I encourage you to follow these steps for the first 30 days as strictly as possible. Since life sometimes gets in the way, I have built in two "cheats" per week. That way, you can stay on the weight-loss track, even while having the occasional indulgence in the first month.

This is not a starvation diet. In fact, you will find you you can choose from many foods both rich in nutrients and light in calories. Remember, the emphasis in the first month is to help you maintain hormonal balance, optimize digestion and be free of cravings. I assure you, after seeing hundreds of people lose anywhere from 10 to 100 pounds, you can do it too!

10 Steps to Re-Setting Your Metabolic Code in 30 Days

1. *Frontload your day.*
2. *Eat protein-rich foods at every meal or snack.*
3. *Eat one serving of high-fiber whole grain per day, preferably at lunch.*
4. *Eat colorful fruits and vegetables throughout your day.*
5. *Eat a sprinkling of good fat.*
6. *Drink eight glasses of water per day.*
7. *Do not drink alcohol for 30 days.*
8. *Pick two treats per week—chocolate, wine or an extra grain.*
9. *Do not eat past 7 p.m.*
10. *Minimize toxic stress.*

1. Frontload Your Day

Do you remember when your mom told you that eating breakfast was the most important meal of the day? Well, it turns out she was right, of course! In addition to picking the right types of foods, research shows that the timing and pacing of meals is also of the utmost importance for weight loss.

Picture your metabolic rate shaped like an ice cream cone. In other words, starting at the top, it is at its highest in the morning and starts to decline on a gradual level as the day progresses. Unfortunately, most of us have a backwards approach to eating when it comes to weight loss and meals. We skip breakfast for a variety of reasons: a lack of hunger, a busy schedule or we want to save on calories. While this may seem to make sense from a pure calories-in, calories-out theory, research has demonstrated time and time again that this approach will result in weight gain. In fact, a study published in *The American Journal of Epidemiology* concluded that skipping meals and eating less frequently translated into weight gain, not weight loss. Consider the following findings:

- Individuals who ate four or more times a day were 45% less likely to be obese than those who ate three times a day or less.
- Skipping breakfast was linked with a greater chance of obesity. People who skipped breakfast were over four times more likely to be obese than those who ate breakfast daily.
- Dining out in restaurants was linked to an increased risk of obesity. This is likely due to the supersizing of portions and to excess saturated fat and calories.

Another research study published in *The European Journal of Clinical Nutrition* showed that skipping meals and irregular meal patterns could decrease insulin sensitivity, thereby promoting weight gain and increasing cardiovascular risk factors. In a nutshell, eating erratically signals the body to burn slower and conserve fat.

In order to lose weight, you need to become a "front loader." In other words, start your day off with a reasonable amount of food. At first, this suggestion may scare breakfast skippers who are not hungry or do not think they have the time to eat. You do not need to eat immediately after you get out of bed; however, you should try to eat your first meal within an hour to an hour and a half of waking for best weight-loss results. You also do not need to eat a huge meal in the morning. A healthy and balanced breakfast of approximately 300 calories is all you need to spark your metabolic engine. I realize that mornings are typically a rushed time, so all the recipe suggestions below can be prepared in under five minutes. In the following chapters, you will be presented with tips and tricks for grocery shopping and staying healthy that, with a little bit of effort in the beginning, will become an easy habit in no time. Here are some examples of breakfasts to front load your day:

Blueberry Yogurt Crunch

Calories = 290

- ½ cup of low fat yogurt
- ½ cup of mixed berries
- 2 tsp. of walnuts sprinkled over top for extra crunch and omega-3!

Combine and enjoy!

Frozen Strawberry Banana Smoothie

Calories = 300

- 5 ounces of soy milk or 1% cow's milk
- ½ frozen banana
- ½ cup of frozen strawberries
- 1 scoop of vanilla protein powder (preferably a whey isolate powder; see product resource guide)
- 1 tsp. flaxseed oil (keep in fridge)

Blend well and enjoy!

Cottage Cheese and Fruit Crunch

Calories = 280

- ½ cup 1% cottage cheese
- ½ cup blueberries
- 4 tbsp. bran cereal
- 1 small banana sliced over top

Combine all ingredients and enjoy!

Cheesy Eggs

Calories = 290

- ½ cup of egg whites
- 1 large omega-3 egg
- 2 ounces grated low-fat cheddar or Swiss cheese
- 1 slice whole grain bread

Add 1 tbsp. of butter to frying pan. Pour in egg whites and omega-3 egg. Add cheese and cook until desired consistency. Enjoy with 1 slice of whole grain bread.

Open-Face Peanut, Almond or Cashew Butter & Banana Sandwich

Calories = 249

- 1 slice omega-3 whole grain bread (see product resource)
- 2 tsp. natural peanut, almond or cashew butter
- ½ sliced banana

Spread peanut butter or substitute on bread, top with sliced bananas and enjoy!

As you will see in the following chapters, in addition to skipping breakfast, high-glycemic and sugar-laden breakfast options such as muffins, instant oatmeal, bagels and refined cereals will leave you feeling sluggish and hungry by approximately 10 or 11 a.m. They will also pack on extra weight. For additional breakfast ideas such as a chocolate lover's smoothie and a Spanish egg white omelet, please refer to the recipe section in the back of the book.

2. Eat Protein-Rich Foods at Every Meal or Snack

Protein is essential for overall health—for muscle repair, hormonal balance, immune system function and for weight loss. Protein also triggers the secretion of a hormone called glucagon which opposes insulin's action and breaks down fat. In other words, the hormones glucagon and insulin are enemies and cannot stand being in the same room with each other! When one is present or up, the other chooses to be down and leaves the room.

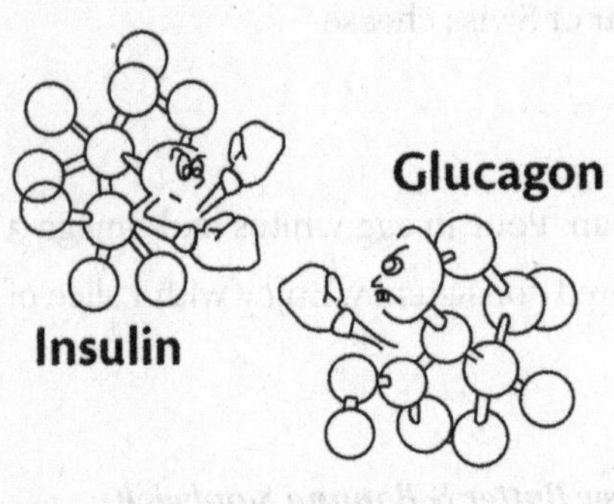

In the nutritional world, we constantly see the rise and fall of various weight-loss fads, popularized through the media and books. The most recent surge was that of the high-protein era—a la Atkins. While the Atkins diet did posses some sound weight-loss advice, there was one major flaw: the body does ***not*** want to use protein as its primary source of fuel. Although the body needs protein, the main source of fuel should come from low-glycemic carbohydrates such as fruits, vegetables, beans and whole grains.

Carbohydrates break down into glucose, a form of sugar that is the primary source of fuel for the body. In fact, protein is quite inefficient as a fuel and when eaten in excess, can put enormous stress on the kidneys. In addition, if you are eating a high-protein diet and are not getting enough sugar in your diet, it can lead to a state called ketosis. Ketosis is a process whereby the body is breaking *itself* down for sugar. This is not an ideal situation—the brain and the body's preferred source of fuel is glucose.

The body can break down muscle and fat into sugar, but it prefers to get it from the low-glycemic index carbohydrates. While some high-protein diets promote and even encourage a state of ketosis, they are not the healthy approach for long-term weight loss. In addition, because proteins need more liquid to be eliminated from the body effectively, the initial weight loss from high-protein diets is usually from water loss, not fat loss. This is why high-protein diets work in the short term: you burn up a lot of fat from glucagon secretion, thereby losing weight and water quickly. However, in a short time you end up feeling sluggish, fatigued and constipated. Even more serious, high-protein diets can potentially lead to detrimental effects on arterial blood flow and kidney function.

There is a fine balance that needs to be struck between the intake of proteins and carbohydrates. Although proteins should not be the mainstay of the diet, they do need to be present at every meal and snack for health and weight-loss purposes. Often times, people who are struggling to lose weight are not eating enough protein. They over-consume the wrong types of carbohydrates, their blood sugar levels bounce around and they have close to zero glucagon secretion.

To begin the first 30 days, you do not have to be too concerned about weighing food or obsessively counting calories. If you follow the 10 steps, you will be in hormonal and caloric balance. What you need to do is to ask yourself the following question at each and every meal or snack: "What is my protein source?" I find that proteins are not as easy to grab as carbohydrates, and therefore, require a little more thought and planning. You do not want the entire meal to be protein, but you do want to have an element of protein in each and every meal.

In addition to protein's hormonal advantage of secreting glucagon and breaking down fat, it is also important to mention the thermic effect of food (TEF). The thermic effect of food refers to the calories you use up daily in digesting the food you eat. This is approximately 10% of all the calories you consume. When it comes to protein, around 25% to 30% of the calories derived from protein are used up in its metabolism. This is significantly higher when compared to 6% to 8% of every 100 calories of carbohydrates and just 2% to 3% of fat. In other words, protein is harder to metabolize and therefore burns more calories. Research has also shown that protein satieties you longer, creating a fuller feeling and causing you to eat less. These are even more reasons to have a good serving of high-quality protein at each and every meal or snack. Remember your new mantra when eating: "What is my protein source?" In order to properly eyeball the amount of protein necessary for weight loss, keep the following in mind: men should strive for 5 to 7 ounces of protein per meal while women should strive for 4 to 6 ounces per meal. The palm of your hand (without fingers or a thumb) or a deck of cards is equivalent to 3 ounces of protein.

Ideal protein options include:

- 4 ounces of chicken (or 1 chicken breast) = 28 grams of protein
- 4 ounces of fish = 28 grams of protein
- 6 ounces (1 can) of tuna = 40 grams of protein
- 4 ounces of lean beef = 28 grams of protein
- 1 large egg = 7 grams of protein
- 1 cup of milk = 8 grams of protein
- 1 ounce of cheese = 7 grams of protein
- ½ cup of cottage cheese = 15 grams of protein
- 1 cup of yogurt = 11 grams of protein
- ½ cup of tofu = 20 grams of protein
- 1 ounce of tofu = 2.3 grams of protein
- 1 cup of soymilk = 6–10 grams of protein
- ½ cup of Tempeh = 15 grams of protein
- ½ cup of lentils cooked = 9 grams of protein
- 1 scoop of protein powder = 15-20 grams of protein

Please note: Most foods contain an element of all three macronutrients which are 1) carbohydrates, 2) proteins, and 3) fats. However, it is the dominant macronutrient that determines the classification of the food. Beans, for instance, contain an element of protein but are higher in carbohydrates and are therefore classified as carbohydrates.

- Most beans (black, pinto, lentils, etc.), ½ cup cooked = approximately 7–10 grams of protein; 15–20 grams of carbohydrates
- Soy beans, ½ cup cooked = 8 grams of protein; 9 grams of carbohydrates
- Split peas, ½ cup cooked = 8 grams of protein; 20 grams of carbohydrates

Nuts and seeds also contain a degree of protein, but are higher in fat and are therefore classified as fats.

- Peanut butter, 2 tablespoons = 8 grams of protein; 17 grams of fat
- Almonds, ¼ cup = 8 grams of protein; 18 grams of fat
- Peanuts, ¼ cup = 9 grams of protein;17 grams of fat
- Cashews, ¼ cup = 5 grams of protein; 15 grams of fat
- Pecans, ¼ cup = 2.5 grams of protein; 17 grams of fat
- Sunflower seeds, 1/2 cup = 6 grams of protein; 12 grams of fat
- Pumpkin seeds, ¼ cup = 9 grams of protein; 12 grams of fat
- Flax seeds, 3 tbsp. = 6 grams of protein; 9 grams of fat

If you are searching for more vegetarian options, nuts and beans can certainly be used to help incorporate more protein into your diet. That said, incorporating some high-quality egg, dairy, fish and poultry options increases variability and offers complete protein sources that will fill you up and trigger glucagon secretion. Here are some easy ways for you to get your daily protein!

Breakfast

- Toast with natural peanut butter
- Protein smoothie
- Scrambled eggs (or egg substitute) with cheese
- Poached egg on whole grain bread

- Yogurt with fruit and nuts
- Protein powder mixed into slow-cooking oatmeal

Lunch

- Turkey slices with veggies and cheese in a sandwich or wrap
- Vegetarian pepperoni sandwich
- Chicken, salmon or tuna salad
- Cottage cheese and fruit
- Spinach salad with chicken and mandarin oranges
- Sliced chicken breast over garden medley salad

Dinner

- Baked or grilled fish (salmon, tuna, tilapia, sole, cod, haddock, halibut, etc.)
- Turkey, chicken or veggie burger
- Stir-fried tofu or chicken with veggies
- BBQ chicken breast
- Salmon patties (see recipe section)
- Chicken, lean beef, turkey or soy meat chili

Snacks

- Yogurt
- Hummus (chickpea dip) with carrots
- Protein bars
- Protein smoothie
- 1 ounce of low-fat cheese with carrots and celery

3. Eat One Serving of High-Fiber Whole Grain per Day, Preferably at Lunch

What's this? Bread is back? In truth, bread was never out. Unfortunately, bread and other grainy carbohydrates were all lumped into the "bad" category, due to the popularity of high-protein diets. With the end of the high-protein era, the research is abundantly clear that whole grain products offer numerous health benefits such as optimizing digestion, reducing cholesterol, preventing cardiovascular disease and even helping with weight loss.

Even with all the positive research on whole grains mounting, nutritional confusion about how to buy the right type of bread still exists. In an attempt to lose weight and keep it off, many people shy away from eating grains altogether. The bottom line is not all grains are created equal! As you will discover in greater detail in Chapter 6, certain grains such as refined flours and sugars cause dramatic blood sugar fluctuations and insulin secretion in the body. Excess insulin secretion promotes the excess storage of fat and will make permanent weight loss almost impossible. This is part of what the first 30 days is protecting you against: sticking to the plan will regulate your hormonal and blood sugar fluctuations making weight loss an easy venture.

In the first 30 days, you can have one serving of high fiber, whole grains per day. I highly recommend having this option at lunch to fill you up and provide you with the perfect energy to continue on with the rest of your day. If you prefer to have your grain at breakfast, that is fine as well. However, it is best to avoid grains at dinner time. The dinner hour should be saved for vegetables and proteins. Here are some examples of grain servings.

- ¾ cup of slow-cooking oatmeal
- 1 slice of whole grain bread (See Product Source Guide)
- ½ cup of whole grain pasta (kamut, spelt)
- ½ cup of brown rice
- 1 small wrap (100% whole wheat or whole grain)

When selecting your grains, ensure that you are buying products labeled "whole grains." I have a lot of confused clients still purchasing "made with whole wheat" who think they are getting whole grain bread. Not necessarily so, my friends. Just because something is listed as whole wheat, does not mean it is made from the whole grain. A whole grain is classified as a product that contains all three parts of the kernel: the bran, the endosperm and the germ. If a grain is refined, it has been stripped of the nutrient-rich bran and germ and only the endosperm, the least nutritious part, remains. In Canada, it is legal to advertise any food product as "whole wheat" even when up to 70% of the germ, a precious part of the grain that contains nutrient value, has been removed. By contrast, in the United States, whole wheat flour contains all three parts of the grain, making it truly a whole grain product.

The best way to get around this labeling debacle is to fight it with proper information. When buying your next loaf of bread, look for bread labeled "whole grain" or which states "100 percent whole wheat" to ensure it contains the germ and the bran. In addition, do not forget your mantra! When you eat your grain selection at lunch, you must match it with a protein of your choice. In other words, your lunch should consist of:

- 1 serving of grain
- 1 selection of protein, approximately 3–5 ounces of tuna, salmon, chicken, turkey slices, egg salad, or veggie meats
- 1 fruit or vegetable servings (or both)

4. Eat Colorful Fruits and Vegetables throughout the Day

We all know that vegetables and fruits are good for us. They are loaded with minerals, vitamins, anti-oxidants and fiber. Most fruits and vegetables are also low on the glycemic index, making them perfect for weight loss and proper blood sugar control. Fruits and vegetables have also been shown to have protective benefits against cancer, heart disease, inflammation, bowel disorders and high cholesterol. Yet, even with all of this powerful information and research, statistics still show that North Americans are not even coming close to meeting their recommended intake per day. Why is this so hard? Where have all the fruit and vegetable eaters gone?

I have found part of the problem is that government agencies, who make the largest dietary recommendations to the public, recommend eating approximately 5 to 10 servings of fruits and vegetables per day. While this is good information, it is hard for most people to visualize this amount of fruits and vegetables, and it rarely translates to their plate. It gets easier when you know what a serving is equivalent to.

Fruits

One serving equals:

- 1 small piece of fruit
- ½ cup raw (cut up) fruit
- ½ cup (4 ounces) of pure, unsweetened fruit juice
- ¼ cup dried fruit
- ½ cup of canned fruit
- ½ of a banana
- 2 small kiwis, apricots or plums

Vegetables

One serving equals:

- 1/2 cup cooked vegetables
- 1 cup raw, leafy vegetables
- 1/2 cup (4 ounces) vegetable juice

Although I do not want you to focus on calories, for general information purposes, a fruit serving is 60 calories and a vegetable serving is 25 calories. As a general rule of thumb, if you eat the right type of calories and are in hormonal balance—the weight will fall off naturally.

In order to clear up any confusion about what and how to eat fruits and vegetables in the next 30 days, let me address a few questions that are likely on your mind.

Can I Eat Too Much Fruit?

Yes, you can. The first 30 days are all about balancing blood sugar, regulating insulin secretion and boosting metabolism. While fruit has enormous health benefits, it can also be slightly higher in sugar and, therefore, intake should be a maximum of 2 servings per day during the next 30 days. Examples for getting more fruit into your diet include:

- Slicing ½ banana over yogurt (1 serving)
- Packing an apple or pear for a snack at work (1 serving)
- Eating ½ cup of blueberries or strawberries stirred into yogurt or cottage cheese (1 serving)
- Using ½ cup of frozen berries or mangos in a morning smoothie (1 serving)
- Using ½ frozen banana in a morning smoothie (1 serving)
- Creating fruit skewers with strawberries, pineapples and grapes (approximately 1 serving) for a healthy and sweet dessert

What about Carrots and Bananas?

Since bananas are a starchier carbohydrate and carrots have a higher glycemic index than other vegetables, certain diets tend to promote totally eliminating them. Even so, the glycemic index of carrots has been tested and re-tested and appears to be significantly lower than once thought. In truth, in all my years of speaking to thousands of people on health and weight loss, I have never met an individual who was struggling with her weight due to eating too many bananas or carrots. In the first month, eating one banana per day (which is equivalent to two servings of fruit) or eating carrots will not tip the scale on weight loss. In other words—go for it. The nutritional value of both of these foods far outweighs the slight increase in sugar. As a general take-home point—pinpointing one or two food items as the obstacle that stands in the way of you reaching your goal weight is unwise. One of my favorite snacks that helps with weight loss and is delicious and filling is hummus (chickpea dip) and carrots. Now, of course, I am not recommending that you eat a large bag of baby carrots and the entire container of hummus! However, 10 baby carrots with 2 tbsp. of hummus will fill you and is the perfect snack.

Can I Have White or Sweet Potatoes?

White potatoes (boiled or mashed) are not allowed as they are high on the glycemic index and tend to trigger the excess storage of fat. Sweet potatoes are starchy, but also possess terrific nutritional benefits such as vitamin C, vitamin A, fiber, iron and potassium, and they are lower on the glycemic index. I do not recommend eating sweet potatoes daily, but having a small sweet potato matched with a protein source one or two times per week is just fine.

Top 10 Anti-Oxidant Vegetables

1. *Broccoli*
2. *Spinach*
3. *Kale*
4. *Green beans*
5. *Beets (steamed or shaved onto salad for color!)*
6. *Carrots*
7. *Squash*
8. *Asparagus*
9. *Peppers*
10. *Artichokes*

Top 10 Anti-Oxidant Fruits

1. *Blueberries*
2. *Blackberries*
3. *Cranberries*
4. *Raspberries*
5. *Strawberries*
6. *Tomatoes*
7. *Apples*
8. *Pears*
9. *Oranges*
10. *Red grapes*

Can I Have Juice?

I always say, "Eat the fruit and drink your water!" By doing so, you will be getting much more fiber per serving of fruit. If you do enjoy juice in your morning shake, in the first 30 days, limit your intake to one cup per day.

In the next 30 days, try to focus on eating fresh foods by including colorful fruits and vegetables throughout your day. Nature is very wise and offers clues about the nutrient value of foods through the vibrancy of their color. Purple, red, green and orange fruits and vegetables are loaded with anti-oxidants and disease-preventing chemicals. As a general rule, try to have two colorful options on your plate per meal.

In terms of vegetables—the more the merrier (with the exception of white potatoes and sweet potatoes). Get as much green food into your system as possible, for example, broccoli, spinach, kale, asparagus and green beans.

Make it your goal to eat a minimum of one citrus fruit and one cruciferous vegetable daily. Less than 10 percent of Americans regularly consume these foods.

5. Eat a Sprinkling of Good Fat

There are three main macronutrients that make up the mainstay of this diet: 1) carbohydrates, 2) proteins and 3) fats. Nature is very wise and provides us with each of these, as they all serve different functions in the body. In fact, all three macronutrients are vital energy sources to the body. Now...I am about to state what should be your second weight-loss mantra. Are you ready? Here we go: any diet that knocks out one of the above three macronutrients or drastically reduces one of them is *not* a sustainable diet! We need fat. In fact, we need all three macronutrients in varying quantities for optimal health, hormonal balance, disease prevention and wellness, and weight loss. If you eliminate one temporarily to lose weight, you will only experience short-term success and often times frustrating weight-loss results.

A great misconception still exists about fats. People tend to shy away from all fats, both good and bad, for fear of excess calories or gaining weight. While it is true that fats contain more than twice the calories of proteins and carbohydrates (carbohydrates and proteins contain 4 calories per gram; fats contain 9 calories per gram), the right type of fat is critical for weight loss, mood control, immune system function and heart health.

Chapter 8 will detail the fats to avoid in your diet in addition to providing information on how to supplement with extra beneficial essential fats. For this section and for the first 30 days, I will detail the fats that are allowed because they are beneficial for hormonal balance and for re-setting your metabolic code.

When thinking of fats, I want you to keep the notion of "sprinkling" top of mind. Simply put, you do not need as much fat as you do proteins and carbohydrates due to the higher amount of calories. That said, indeed you do require fats daily and can easily fit them into most meals and snacks. The mainstay of fats should be derived from monounsaturated fats and omega-3 fats.

Monounsaturated Fats

A high consumption of monounsaturated fats such as olive oil is thought to be one of the reasons that Mediterranean countries have one of the lowest rates of heart disease in the world. These fats also appear to lower total cholesterol and LDL (the "bad" cholesterol) and increase HDL (the "good" cholesterol). In terms of weight loss, research in *The British Journal of Clinical Nutrition* demonstrated that simply switching saturated fats, e.g., full fat cheeses and red meats, for monounsaturated fats caused obese patients to lose a significant amount of weight. Even though the calories were exactly the same, monounsaturated fats such as olive oil appeared to have positive fat-burning effects. This is even more evidence that re-setting your metabolic code takes more than a calories-in, calories-out approach. Your quality of food choices, which is tied in with maintaining hormonal balance, is equally as powerful and necessary for successful and permanent weight loss as is counting calories.

Monounsaturated fats are found in natural foods such as avocados and nuts and they are the main component of olive oil (75%) and canola oil (57%–60%). Olive oil is the best fat for cooking and has the highest oxidation threshold. In other words, it remains stable at high temperatures for a long time without becoming rancid. When selecting olive oil, purchase cold pressed extra virgin olive oil made from the first pressing of the olive. Store your olive oil in a dark, cool environment and use within the first few months of purchasing.

Essential Fats

There are two types of polyunsaturated fats that are called essential fatty acids. In other words, these fats are essential to life and must come from the diet as the body cannot make them.

1. Linoleic acid (LA) is an omega-6 fatty acid found in vegetables oils such as corn safflower, soybean and sunflower oil as well as primrose and borage oil.

2. Alpha-linolenic (ALA) is an omega-3 fatty acid found in flaxseed oil, flaxseeds, hemp, sesame seeds, walnuts, almonds, green leafy vegetables and blueberries. The body converts ALA into the longer chain fatty acids eicosapentaenoic acid (EPA) and docosahexaenoic acid (DHA) also found in cold water fish, e.g., salmon, tuna, halibut and herring, and fish oil.

Linoleic (LA) acid is (omega-6) plentiful in the diet and deficiencies rarely occur. In fact, eating too much LA in the form of refined vegetable oils can result in inflammation and a fatty liver. More commonly, people are deficient in ALA—omega-3 fat and its derivatives DHA and EPA. DHA and EPA have been shown to protect against heart disease, aid in proper brain function and act as an anti-inflammatory agent (for more on essential fats, see Chapter 8). For weight loss, omega-3 fats have also been shown to increase fat loss. Studies have demonstrated that adding fish oil supplements (an omega-3 source) to the diet in replacement of saturated fats also promotes significant weight loss in terms of abdominal fat and overall body mass index (BMI).

In a nutshell, the above mentioned types of fat can actually help you lose weight and feel better. However, the key point is—don't over do it! The following recommended serving sizes of fats can be used in your meals for the first 30 days.

- 1–2 tbsp. of olive oil for sautéing vegetables or other foods. You can dress up a salad with the second tablespoon of oil and some lemon juice or balsamic vinegar.
- 8–10 nuts such as almonds or walnuts
- ¼ of an avocado on a salad or in a sandwich or wrap
- 1–2 tbsp. of flaxseed oil in a dressing over a salad
- 2 tbsp. of toasted sesame seeds over a salad or on chicken
- 1tsp. of canola oil or olive oil to make your morning eggs
- 1 tbsp. of ground flaxseeds over salad, in a morning shake, or in a yogurt snack.

Note: Never heat flaxseed oil as it can damage the oil. Store flaxseed oil and flaxseeds in the fridge. If grinding flaxseeds, store them in an air-tight, opaque container and discard after 90 days. Once you grind flax-seed, there is a greater risk of it developing an off-flavor and taste. Ideally, it is best to grind whole flaxseeds and to use them immediately.

6. Drink Eight Glasses of Water per Day

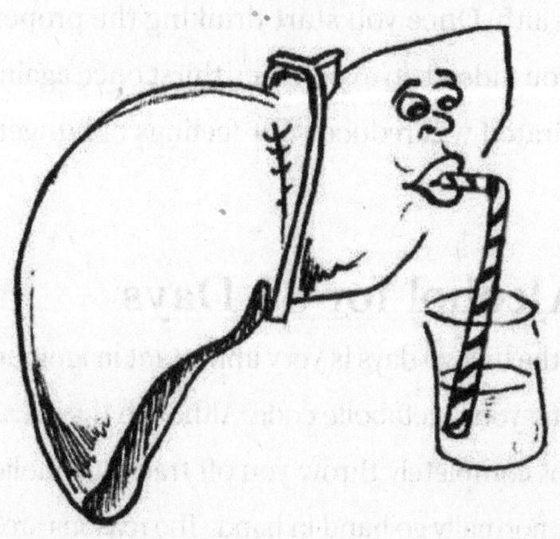

Similar to food, lack of water can also slow the metabolic rate. How can that be, you ask. Water is partially involved with the functioning of your liver. Part of the liver's duty is to break down and metabolize fat. However, if the liver receives a message that the kidneys are water deprived, it picks up the slack of the kidneys and turns its concentration to water retention instead of burning fat. In other words, in addition to taxing the liver, being in a state of dehydration will also promote fat storage.

How Much Water Is Enough?

Eight 8-ounce glasses per day is optimal for weight loss, proper digestive functioning and extra energy. If this sounds like a lot, keep in mind you do not need to drink all of this water at once. Try to spread your water consumption throughout the day. For example, select three to four times a day to drink a glass of water and try to take sips in between those times. In addition, adding a slice of lemon or lime, drinking herbal teas or adding a small amount of natural juice (¼ glass of juice with ¾ glass of water) will also help to hydrate your system.

During the first few days of increasing your water consumption, you may be running to the bathroom a little more than usual. This is a complaint I often encounter. Take heed; this is quite normal and will soon pass. What is occurring is actually a very positive thing. After finally receiving proper hydration, the body is flushing itself. In other words, your system will let go of the water it has been holding on to for survival and replace it with the water you are now drinking.

The other common complaint I often hear is "I am not thirsty!" If you are not thirsty, you are already dehydrated. Thirst and hunger are normal sensations that are a sign of health. Once you start drinking the proper amount of water, you will find you indeed do experience thirst once again. In addition, being properly hydrated will reduce your feelings of hunger, causing you to eat less.

7. Do Not Drink Alcohol for 30 Days

The avoidance of alcohol during the first 30 days is very important in igniting the metabolic flame and re-setting your metabolic code. Although the occasional alcoholic beverage will not completely throw you off track, alcoholic beverages and weight loss do not normally go hand in hand. The reasons are:

- Fat metabolism can decrease by as much as a whopping 73% for several hours after having a drink.
- Having a drink before or with a meal causes you to consume 200 calories or more without your even realizing it!

Additional research on alcohol also demonstrates that the body burns up the calories from alcohol first, leaving the others to be converted and stored as fat.

For some, eliminating alcohol from the diet for 30 days is an easy step—a "no-brainer," as someone in my practice recently told me. For others who enjoy a daily drink, this step (similar to cutting back on coffee) can often be more challenging. If you are someone who enjoys a glass or two of red wine daily, do not panic. As you will see in the following step, you are allowed a certain number of cheats per week. By doing so, you will avoid feelings of deprivation and/or restriction and will still be able to continue on the weight-loss track.

8. Pick Two Treats per Week—Chocolate, Wine or an Extra Grain

What's this? Treats on a weight-loss program? After years of working with people who need to lose weight, I have found the key to long-term success is to have enough foods that balance hormones in controlled portion sizes combined with real-life options and the occasional treat. In other words, if the plan is not realistic for most of us who lead busy lives, we will not follow through. Of course, getting healthy and losing weight does take more focus, time and commitment, but it can also be fun and enjoyable!

Trust me, occasional treats are *not* the reason we have an obesity epidemic in North America. When you look at the statistics—more than one out of every four children is overweight or obese and more than six out of every 10 adults are overweight or obese—you quickly realize much more is going on. The reason that more than half of us are overweight has more to do with increased portion sizes, lack of exercise, eating too many refined flours and sugars, and the onslaught of fast food. Top that off with stress, lack of sleep and a go, go, go lifestyle and presto—5, 10, 15 pounds quickly turns into more and increases our disease risk dramatically.

When selecting your two treats per week, you will find the treat list includes healthier versions of treats. You did not actually think I was going to recommend eating white refined flour cookies or trans fat-filled doughnuts did you? That said, I ask you to take my treat challenge. I promise you they will taste equally delicious and satisfying as your old goodies. By allowing yourself to indulge in the treats outlined below twice per week, you will curb cravings and will also keep on the 30-day track to re-setting your metabolic code.

Treats that are allowed two times per week during the first 30 days include:

Red wine If indulging in alcohol, make it red wine. With its cardio-protective benefit and only 80 calories per glass, it is a much better option than hard alcohol (vodka or gin) or beer. During the first 30 days, you can have up to two 4-ounce glasses per week.

Extra dark chocolate The celebrated French physician Francis Joseph Victor Broussais put it best when he said, "Chocolate of good quality...calms the fever, nourishes the patient and tends to restore him to health." When recent research demonstrated that dark chocolate was indeed good for overall health, chocolate lovers all over the world celebrated! The good news is that dark chocolate contains an abundant amount of anti-oxidants that appear to help lower blood pressure and may even be beneficial for diabetes and blood sugar control. The benefits appear to come from the plant phenols, especifically the cocoa phenols that are found in dark chocolate.

So...while I am not licensing you to go on a chocolate binge, it is okay to indulge up to twice a week on dark chocolate in moderation. What is moderation? I recommend purchasing a large chocolate bar made with 70% cocoa and chopping it up into small squares. Allow yourself to have three small squares as a treat two times per week.

Extra serving of grain In the first 30 days, it is important to regulate and limit grain in order to balance insulin secretion and increase metabolic function. In the following chapters on carbohydrates and proteins, you will discover in detail why striking a balance between the hormones insulin and glucagon is of the utmost importance for weight loss, energy and disease prevention.

For the first 30 days, you are allowed to eat one grain per day. Extra grain treats could include:

- ¾ cup of slow-cooking oatmeal
- 1 slice of whole grain bread
- ½ cup of whole grain pasta (kamut, spelt)
- ½ cup of brown rice
- 1 wrap (100% whole wheat or whole grain)

Remember, it is best to eat your grain option at breakfast or lunch. Dinnertime should be reserved for protein and vegetables. In addition—I cannot stress this enough—only go for whole-grain options.

9. Do Not Eat Past 7 p.m.

When considering the calories-in, calories-out theory of weight loss, the time of day a meal is eaten should not make a difference. However, I can tell you from years of working with weight-loss success stories (myself included after gaining 70 pounds while pregnant), it definitely makes a difference!

There are several reasons as to why late-night eaters gain more weight. First, late-night eating is often a time when people are tired at the end of a long day; they are feeling more emotional and are craving starch. Instead of eating protein and vegetables, which takes more planning and focus, they quickly eat a large amount of the wrong food choices such as a big plate of pasta, pizza, a sub or even a bowl of cereal if they feel lazy! Late-night snacking is a big issue for most people. When feeling hungry and experiencing cravings due to being out of hormonal balance, mindless eating sets in (usually in front of the TV) and unconscious munching on crackers, cookies, cereal, chocolate, fruit and bread occurs. The result? An over secretion of the hormone insulin, which promotes the storage of fat.

In addition to weight gain, late-night eating can also compromise digestion and energy. Your body does not want to be digesting a huge amount of food late at night. This is not the time when your metabolic engine is strongest. According to Ayurvedic medicine, an ancient system of health care that is native to the Indian subcontinent, it is best to eat the largest meal of the day at lunch, between 12 and 1 p.m., when digestion is strongest.

While it is true that there is not much research into the fact that late-night eating helps with weight loss and digestion, I can tell you from clinical experience, unless you are diabetic, it works each and every time. While research into diet and natural health is growing at a rapid pace, more research is warranted. On the subject of late night eating and weight gain.

Ideally, during the first 30 days, a typical day should resemble the following meal schedule:

Breakfast (7–8 a.m.)

- 1 serving of fruit
- 1 serving of protein (1 scoop of protein powder, ½ cup cottage cheese or yogurt, ¼ cup of egg whites mixed with one egg)
- Sprinkle of fat (t tbsp. of ground flaxseeds or flaxseed oil)

Lunch (12–1 p.m.)

- 1 serving of grain (i.e. 1 slice of bread)
- 1 serving of protein (tuna, salmon, chicken, turkey slices, egg salad, veggie meats – 4-6 ounces)
- 1 fruit or vegetable serving (or both)

Snack (3–4 p.m.) (choose one from the list below)

- 1 vegetable serving with 1 ounce of low fat cheese
- 8–10 nuts

- Protein bar
- 1 serving of yogurt
- 1 serving of hummus and carrots
- 1 ounce of cheese and sliced apples

Dinner (6–7 p.m.)

- 1 protein serving (4-6 ounces)
- 2 servings of vegetables
- Sprinkle of fat (1 tbsp. of olive oil, canola oil, or ¼ of an avocado sliced)

People often find not eating late at night one of the hardest steps to follow. People who work late or do shift work find this step nearly impossible. These concerns are real and need to be addressed. First, if you are working late at the office, try to pack your dinner and eat it by 7 p.m. Alternatively, if you are ordering in, keep your intake to vegetables and protein. If you know you are pulling an "all nighter" pack some fruit, yogurt and water to keep your energy up. If on most nights you meet the 7 p.m. rule and you fall off occasionally due to business, holidays etc., you are doing great.

If you are working shift work, i.e., overnight, this is a tough one. You will need to eat throughout your shift to keep your energy up and weight down. This is all the more reason to focus on low-glycemic index carbohydrates such as fruits and vegetables, lean proteins such as yogurt, turkey slices and protein bars, and essential fats such as raw almonds, walnuts, and seeds (i.e., sunflower or pumpkin seeds).

In short, the body thrives on a daily schedule and routine. By eating breakfast, lunch, dinner and one snack per day, you will keep your metabolic engine humming 24 hours per day, seven days per week. To quote Adele Davis, an American pioneer in the field of nutrition, "Eat Breakfast like a king, lunch like a prince, and dinner like a pauper."

10. Minimize Emotional Toxins

In the year 2007, we have more access to each other and global information than at any previous time in history. Blackberries, cell phones, fax machines, email, you name it, we are constantly stimulated. With all of our responsibilities and workload, North Americans are more stressed than ever. Prescription medications for anxiety and panic disorders such as lorazepam (brand name Ativan) are also being prescribed at an all-time high.

The majority of North Americans are walking around with a high degree of stress, often without realizing it, and the toll it takes on physical and mental health is enormous.

When I first see a client, as part of the health history I ask the client to rate his or her daily level of stress. Ten represents unbearable stress and 0 represents no stress at all. The common response is 7 or 8 out of 10. That is quite high!

Whether derived from something personal, financial, your family, work or relationships, mild to moderate chronic stress can greatly hinder your health and promote weight gain. When your body perceives it is stressed, your brain releases chemicals to help your body handle the situation and respond with the appropriate physical response. This response has been termed the "fight or flight" response. Although this is a necessary and appropriate short-term response, when the stress becomes chronic and the switch on the fight-or-flight response does not shut off, a myriad of reactions can occur in your body that can lead to weight gain.

During times of stress, the body secretes a hormone called cortisol, otherwise known as the stress hormone. An over-secretion of cortisol promotes weight gain in a number of ways.

- **Lowered metabolism** Too much cortisol can slow your metabolism, causing more weight gain than you would normally experience.
- **Increased food cravings** People who are over-secreting cortisol tend to crave more salty and sweet foods such as candy, ice cream, cookies, potato chips, etc.
- **Blood sugar irregularities** Prolonged stress and cortisol secretion

causes fluctuations in blood sugar levels, creating feelings of fatigue, moodiness and mental fogginess.

- **Fat storage** Certain studies show that elevated cortisol tends to cause weight gain around the abdominal area vs. the hips. This type of fat deposition is called "toxic fat" because it is strongly correlated with the development of heart disease and stroke.

Exercise: The Stress Buster

The most effective way to lower cortisol levels, decrease stress, boost metabolism and lose weight is to exercise. During the first 30 days and after, you need to implement some sort of exercise into your daily regime a minimum of five times per week. Of those five times, three should consist of a minimum of 30-minute cardiovascular workouts (treadmill, brisk walking, running, racquet sports, elliptical) and two workouts should include weights for both upper and lower body. You also need to do abdominal work (sit-ups) five times per week.

Yoga is also a wonderful discipline for stress management and helps to open up and elongate the joints, and Pilates is fantastic for developing core strength. If you cannot make it to a class or a local community center due to your schedule, there are a variety of yoga and Pilates DVDs and CDs available that you can use in the privacy of your own home.

It is also of the utmost importance to implement stress management techniques into your daily life. These do not take long, but they can dramatically affect the way you feel.

- If you are an office worker sitting at your desk all day, stand up every 40–60 minutes, clasp your hands behind your back and extend your spine to stretch. This and this alone will give you a little energy boost.
- Belly breath. If you are feeling a sense of stress or panic, inhale for the count of five through your nose while your belly expands, exhale for a count of five and let your belly drop. Most people are "upper chest breathers" when stressed. Belly breathing switches your body

from a sympathetic "fight or flight" response to the opposite, called a parasympathetic response. In other words, it is nearly impossible to have a panic attack or feel stressed at the same time you are belly breathing!

- Take the stairs whenever you can. My motto is, as long as you can walk the stairs, you should!
- Watch caffeine intake. More than one cup of coffee per day can cause jitters, irritation and feelings of being on a short fuse. Herbal teas, green or white tea can help hydrate the system and are very helpful for weight loss.
- Journal nightly. Writing your thoughts, goals and feelings on paper has a magical effect. Not only does it help to de-stress the mind and body, it will help keep you focused on the direction you wish to go. Try it—it works!
- Do not overdo it with the media. We are constantly bombarded with imagery of war, bombings, murders, etc. Without even realizing it, this has an enormous effect on our psyche and stress levels. If you are a sports fan, enjoy music and have a certain show that helps to de-stress you, by all means, enjoy it for the half-hour or hour. Keep in mind, though, it is best not to be bombarded with negative news messages and images throughout your day, especially before bed.
- Strike your own balance. This is easier said than done and means something different to every individual. For me, eating well and exercising is the best way to help me be a better mother, wife, writer, etc. Although some refined floury treats may taste good temporarily, the way they make me feel afterwards is just not worth it. As I always say, "We do better when we feel better!"

Now that you have been introduced to and understand the 10 steps to re-setting your metabolic code, you are ready to begin. Try to stick to these guidelines as strictly as possible for the first month, and you will begin to see the pounds melt away. Even more important, you will be revving your metabolic engine and setting the stage for hormonal balance for life! The next chapter details more tips and tricks for the first 30 days.

Marianne

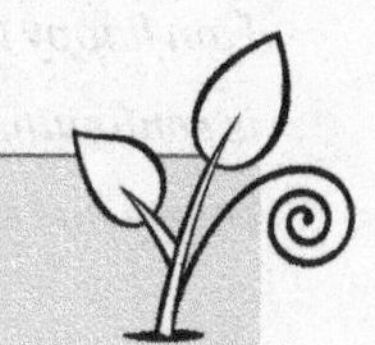

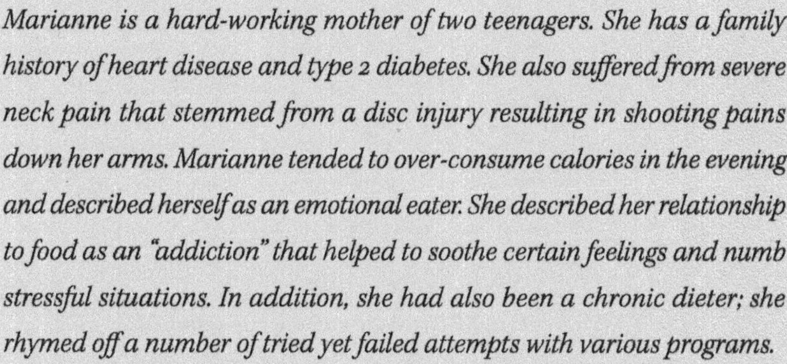

Height: *5 feet 4 inches*

Weight: *226 pounds*

Goal weight: *150–160 pounds*

Current BMI: *38.8*

Total weight loss: *42 pounds and still losing!*

Marianne is a hard-working mother of two teenagers. She has a family history of heart disease and type 2 diabetes. She also suffered from severe neck pain that stemmed from a disc injury resulting in shooting pains down her arms. Marianne tended to over-consume calories in the evening and described herself as an emotional eater. She described her relationship to food as an "addiction" that helped to soothe certain feelings and numb stressful situations. In addition, she had also been a chronic dieter; she rhymed off a number of tried yet failed attempts with various programs.

At our first meeting, Marianne struck me as a very kind and upbeat individual. Yet, she also told me she was a constant "doer" for others and always put herself at the end of her list. Her openness and newly attained attitude of "I need to do this for me" set the perfect stage for her to regain control of her weight and health. She had recently returned to the workforce after 17 years spent raising her children and was taking specific steps to implement order into her life. Unfortunately, due to faulty food choices, Marianne lacked the energy she needed throughout the day. Upon reviewing Marianne's food intake, it was obvious why she was gaining weight and experiencing varying levels of fatigue. Her entire day consisted of foods that were going to put her into an insulin/blood-sugar roller coaster. Her protein intake was low and her intake of high-glycemic index choices such as bagels, banana bread, white pasta and processed crackers was high. Due to the fluctuations in her blood sugar and insulin levels, if Marianne skipped a meal, she would feel shaky and experience intense cravings.

After implementing the steps to re-setting her metabolic code (it took her 60 days instead of 30) and adding in three to four workouts per week, I am happy to report that Marianne has lost 42 pounds and 23 inches and is continuing to lose! Her neck pain has improved tremendously and her energy has soared.

5

Tips and Tricks for Re-Setting Your Metabolic Code

"If I'd known I was gonna live this long. I'd have taken better care of myself!"

Eubie Blake, (1883-1983)
American song writer and composer at 100 years old

As you now know, your metabolism plays a significant role in weight management: the faster your metabolism, the more calories you will burn, and the less likely that you will be overweight. This chapter will provide you will all the tools and knowledge you will need to effectively spark the flame on your metabolic engine in the first 30 days and to stay on track.

Your 30-Day Grocery Cart

To make life easier (and who doesn't want that?), it is important to stock up on some core items during the first 30 days. Before starting, I highly recommend taking the list below to your local grocery or health food store and making sure you have all the food tools to lose weight. Your 30-day grocery shop does not have to be an expensive venture, but it is necessary to fill your fridge and cupboards with the basics you will need.

In addition to the grocery list below, prior to beginning your 30 days, you need to do a complete kitchen audit. In other words, open up your cupboards and fridge, and eliminate the bad. Processed crackers, cereals, candy, pop, cookies, chocolate bars, white bread and pasta need to be thrown out or given away. If you have children who tend to eat junk, instead of removing it all at once, I highly recommend gradually directing them towards healthier food choices. Kids learn by example. When they see Mom or Dad eating healthy and delicious food, they will soon partake and enjoy it as well. If junk food is not available and accessible in your kitchen, it is better for the entire family.

Your 30-day grocery cart should contain the following foods.

Carbohydrates

- All vegetables, with the exception of white potatoes. Emphasis should be on green vegetables such as broccoli, kale, rapini, and spinach and on red tomatoes and tomato sauce. Cucumbers, bok choy, celery, baby carrots and cut up peppers are also great options when you want a crunchy snack.

- All fruits, with the exception of dates, lychee nuts and raisins. Emphasis should be on berries (strawberries, raspberries and blueberries), apples, peaches, plums and oranges. Bags of mixed frozen berries are available at most grocery stores. These are great for morning shakes.
- Beans—navy beans, chickpeas, black beans, lima beans, garbanzo beans, kidney beans, hummus (chickpea) dip. (Remember, beans are a good source of protein as well.)
- Whole-grain bread (See product resource section for recommendations).
- Brown rice or brown basmati rice (Avoid all instant rice).
- Kamut, spelt or whole grain pasta. Cook your pasta el dente (under cook by 1-2 minutes) to lower glycemic index value.

Note: Whenever possible, buy 100% certified organic produce. Food that is approved with organic 100% certification is free of herbicide, fungicide or pesticide residue. The more toxicity you can reduce in your body—the better!

Proteins

- Sole
- Halibut
- Mackerel
- Tilapia
- Haddock
- Canned tuna (light)
- Canned salmon
- Salmon fillet
- Sardines
- Cartons of egg whites
- Omega-3 eggs

- Low-fat yogurt
- Low-fat or 1% cottage cheese
- Low-fat cream cheese
- Skim or low-fat milk
- Soy milk
- Turkey breast
- Turkey slices
- Chicken breast
- Chicken slices
- Tempeh
- Tofu
- Vegetarian burgers
- Edamame
- Lean beef
- Protein powder (whey isolate)

Note: If you are a vegetarian, you will need to incorporate some sort of protein option into your diet such as soy, dairy, rice or egg protein.

Fats

- Ripe avocados
- Walnuts
- Almonds
- Natural nut butters (almond, peanut, cashew)
- Flaxseeds (golden or brown)
- Flaxseed oil (keep in fridge)
- Extra virgin olive oil
- Olives—black or green (6 maximum at a time)
- Canola oil
- Sesame seeds
- Pumpkin seeds

Note: You will also get some essential omega-3 fat from eating the cold water fish (salmon or tuna) recommended above.

Treats and Additional Items

- Dark chocolate (65–70% cocoa)
- Red wine
- Green tea
- White tea
- Balsamic vinaigrette for salad dressings
- Flavorings for food—mustard, garlic, herbs (e.g., fresh basil, coriander, dill)
- Bean dips such as black bean dips or hummus
- Popcorn kernels for air-popped popcorn

Some Common Questions and Answers about Foods

After stocking up on all the delicious and tasty food options to keep you on track—you will be perfectly set up to rev your metabolic engine in the first 30 days. You may have some questions while going thru the first month about specific foods. If so, simply refer to the questions and answers provided below to fill in any gaps.

Question: Should I drink green, white or black tea?

Answer: All three! Green tea and white tea are both made from the same plant (the Camellia sinensis plant), although they have undergone different processing. Green tea is a lightly processed tea that is not fermented. The leaf is either baked, roasted, sun dried or steamed after harvesting to stop the fermentation process. When the leaves are sufficiently dried, they are rolled into a variety of shapes. For weight loss, green tea contains high concentrations of catechin polyphenols. These compounds work in the body with other chemicals to heighten levels of fat oxidation and thermogenesis (a state created in the body by burning fat as fuel). On average, you should try to consume a minimum of three cups of green tea per day for its weight-loss effect. Green tea has also been shown to be preventative against cancer, heart disease and high cholesterol. Current studies demonstrate green tea to be an anti-stress beverage. Green tea contains the amino acid called L-theanine that helps to lower the stress response.

White tea leaves are the least processed and are picked and harvested while the leaf is still in bud form. The buds are covered with fine white hair giving the tea its white look. Although similar to green tea, white tea does not have the same "grassy" taste and contains more of a light sweet flavor. In terms of health, white tea has been shown to contain even greater anti-oxidant capacity than green tea, and studies have shown white tea to have a potent anti-bacterial, anti-viral effect. Although terrific for overall health, the effects of white tea and weight loss have not been documented. I recommend you consume a mixture of green and white tea throughout the day.

Black tea is also been made from the same plant as white and green tea (the Camellia sinensis plant), but has been fully processed and fermented. Although further research is warranted, preliminary studies indicate that drinking black tea can be beneficial for prevention of stroke and heart disease. If you are a black tea lover, I recommend consuming one cup per day in addition to white and green teas.

Question: What is Edamame? Is it a source of protein?

Answer: Edamame is a green vegetable known as a soybean. In East Asia, the soybean has been used as a major source of protein for over 2000 years. Edamame can be used as the perfect low-calorie, high-protein snack instead of crackers, chips or cookies. In our house, we make a big bowl of Edamame with sea salt to munch on when watching a movie.

How to cook Edamame: To retain freshness, Edamame is typically parboiled and quick frozen. It can be found in the freezer section of most health food stores or Asian markets. To prepare, simply boil the pods in unsalted water for 10 minutes. Shell the beans inside simply by squeezing the pods with your fingers or mouth. You can also add some sea salt for taste.

Question: What is tempeh?

Answer: For those who equate tofu with bland, tasteless cubes, you will be happy to learn about tempeh. Tempeh is made from cooked and fermented soybeans that are formed into a patty. It has a similar protein and calcium content as tofu, and it also contains the beneficial isoflavones (anti-oxidant compounds that have anti-cancer properties) of tofu. Tempeh has a wonderful nutty flavor and texture. It can be added into stir-fries, soups or chili. It can be on the dry side if not seasoned properly, so adding sauce for moisture is recommended. Tempeh is available in the freezer section of most health food stores.

Tips and Tricks in the Grocery Store and Beyond

- Go for bulk. Your bulk food section contains a variety of healthy snack foods such as walnuts, almonds and dried apples. Check nuts for smell and taste when purchasing, and store them in the fridge whenever possible. Ask the staff how long they have been sitting in the containers. Nuts can easily go bad due to their precious oil content. You can purchase shelled or unshelled nuts. Unshelled nuts have a longer shelf life, but also take more time to prepare. I purchase and enjoy unshelled raw almonds or walnuts on a weekly basis as part of my "healthy fat" options. Bulk spices and whole grains are also available.
- Get an organic delivery box. In addition, familiarize yourself with local organic markets that may be open in your area, visit local farmers' markets and check out your usual grocery stores. Many now offer high-quality organic produce.
- Consider putting a water purification system in your home or invest

in a monthly water dispenser unit. Reverse osmosis and distilled water are excellent choices. Having water easily accessible in your home will encourage you to drink more and will boost your metabolism.

- For a summertime sweet treat, purchase Popsicle makers and make your own healthy Popsicles. See the shake recipes in recipe section in the back of the book. Simply prepare and freeze. Remember, Popsicle treats are not just for the kids!
- If you have the freezer space, stock up on protein options such as chicken breasts, wild salmon fillets and veggie burgers. It is a good idea to always have easy-to-grab protein options in your home.
- Put oil in a spray can and spray it on fruits and vegetables. You can even invest in some deliciously seasoned olive oils.
- Get to know your health food stores. Take an hour to walk up and down the aisles of your local health food store or the natural value section of your local grocery store.
- Invest in a good blender. It is a must for a healthy home and can be used to make morning protein smoothies, puréed soups and bean dips such as hummus.
- Create meals on Sundays. Use Sunday as the day to grocery shop and plan healthy meals for the week. You can freeze homemade soups, chilis or stews. This is also a great time to stock up on vegetables, fruits and bulk food options. Cut up your veggies when you are home (i.e. celery, broccoli florets, etc.). So you have grab-and-go easy snack options.
- Cut fresh lemon into slices and keep them in the fridge. When drinking a glass of water, add a lemon slice for taste and for the natural astringent effect it has on digestion.

Sample Meal Plans

Following you will find one week of recommended meal plans. If you do not like a specific meal suggestion, simply skip it. This is to give you ideas on how and what to eat during the first month. Keep in mind that eating well and losing weight requires a bit of a learning curve. I have found many of the people I see in practice are creatures of habit, and initially they prefer eating the same thing over and over when the pounds first start falling off. When losing my baby weight, I too had a similar theme in the meals I was eating on a daily basis. You will find once the routine starts to work for you and you feel more confident in your ability to lose, you will start experimenting with different healthy food choices.

If you do enjoy a lot of daily variety in your food choices, the meal plans and the recipes throughout and at the back of this book (in the recipe section) will provide you with plenty of options. Get creative! You can enjoy a whole spectrum of delicious foods and tastes when you delve into the world of healthy eating.

Note: If you would like to switch your afternoon snack to a morning snack between breakfast and lunch that is fine. However, all the breakfasts should have enough protein and fat to keep you energized and satisfied until lunchtime.

Monday

Breakfast: ***Mixed Berry Shake (serves 1)***

- 1 scoop protein powder
- 4 ounces water
- 4 ounces orange juice
- ½ cup frozen berries (mixed frozen berries)
- 1 tsp. flaxseed oil or ground flaxseeds

Simply add all ingredients to your blender. Blend on high for 2 minutes and enjoy!

Lunch: ***Lox and Cream Cheese with Fruit (serves 1)***

- 1 slice whole-grain bread
- 2 tsps. light cream cheese
- 4 ounces smoked salmon
- 1 piece of fruit (1 small apple, peach, plum, pear or 2 Clementine oranges)
- Carrots and celery

Spread cream cheese on whole grain bread and top with 5 ounces of smoked salmon (wild salmon if possible). Enjoy with piece of fruit and vegetables on the side.

Snack

- 1 small yogurt (4 ounces, any flavor, naturally sweetened)

Dinner: ***Lemon-Roasted Salmon (serves 4)***

- 4 tbsp. lemon juice
- 2 tsp. extra virgin olive oil
- ½ tsp. black pepper
- 1 ½ pound salmon fillet, in one piece, skin on

- ½ tsp. salt
- 2 tbsp. capers
- 6 slices of fresh lemon

Preheat oven to 425°F. Brush a cooking sheet with extra virgin olive oil. Place the salmon, skin-side down, on the baking sheet. Rub the olive oil onto the salmon and sprinkle with the salt and pepper. Distribute the lemon juice over the fillet. Sprinkle the capers over top and cover fillet with 6 lemon slices. Bake for 25 minutes or until the salmon is medium-done. Lift the salmon off the baking sheet, leaving the skin behind. Enjoy with side salad.

Tuesday

Breakfast: ***Chocolate Banana Smoothie (Serves 1)***

- 8 ounces soy milk or low-fat milk
- 1 scoop chocolate protein powder
- ½ medium-sized banana (frozen)
- 2 tsp. ground flaxseeds or flaxseed oil
- 1 tsp. chocolate syrup

Simply add all ingredients to your blender. Blend on high for 2 minutes and enjoy!

Lunch: ***Mediterranean Pizza (Serves 4)***

- 1 whole-grain pizza crust (available in most health food and grocery stores
- ½ cup of tomato sauce
- 1 garlic clove, finely chopped
- 1 cup shredded chicken
- ½ cup sliced green or black olives
- ½ tsp. dried oregano
- ½ tsp. dried basil
- 1 cup reduced-fat cheese (mozzarella and/or cheddar blend)

Preheat oven to 450°F. Spread tomato sauce over the crust. Sprinkle toppings on pizza, finishing with cheese. Bake on a pizza sheet or pizza stone for 10 minutes. Enjoy 2 slices for lunch with a side salad.

Note: This pizza can be pre-made and taken to the office or school for a healthy and delicious lunch for the entire family.

Snack

- Carrots, cucumbers, celery and 2 tsp. of hummus

Dinner: ***Spinach Salad with Grilled Chicken Breast and Avocado (Serves 1)***

- 4 ounces roasted or grilled chicken breast chopped into small cubes
- 2 cups baby leaf spinach
- 2 tsp. balsamic vinaigrette
- 2 plum tomatoes, sliced
- ¼ avocado, thinly sliced
- 1 apple, on the side

Add baby spinach and tomatoes to a serving bowl. Top with sliced avocado and cubed roasted chicken breast. Toss with balsamic vinaigrette and enjoy with apple on the side.

Wednesday

Breakfast: ***Anti-Aging Smoothie (Serves 1)***

- 4 ounces orange juice
- 1 scoop protein powder
- 4 ounces water and/or crushed ice
- ¼ cup frozen mango
- ¼ cup blueberries
- 2 tsp. ground flaxseeds or flaxseed oil

Simply add all ingredients to your blender. Blend on high for 2 minutes and enjoy!

Lunch: ***Turkey wrap (Serves 1)***

- 1 whole-wheat wrap
- 4 ounces turkey breast, sliced
- 1 ounce low-fat cheese, Cheddar or Swiss
- 3 tbsp. Lettuce
- 3 tbsp. of diced tomatoes
- ½ handful almonds, on the side
- 1 tsp. low-fat honey mustard dressing

Place sliced turkey in wrap, add in cheese (shred if desired), tomato, lettuce and honey mustard dressing. Fold wrap and enjoy with almonds on the side.

Snack

- 1 apple
- 1 ounce low-fat cheese

Dinner: ***Chicken and/or Tofu Stir-Fry with Mixed Vegetables (Serves 1)***

- 6 ounces boneless chicken breast or 6 ounces extra firm tofu, seasoned
- ½ head broccoli, chopped
- ½ cup water chestnuts,
- ½ cup celery, chopped
- ½ onion, chopped
- ½ red pepper, diced
- 1 tsp. olive oil
- 1 tsp. minced ginger
- 2 tbsp. soy sauce

Slice chicken or tofu thinly. Use 1 tsp. of olive oil in fry pan. Combine all ingredients including 1 tsp. minced ginger and 1 tbsp. Soy sauce. Cover and cook on medium high heat until vegetables are cooked but still crunchy.

Thursday

Breakfast: ***Creamy Strawberry Smoothie (Serves 1)***

- 5 ounces soy milk or low-fat milk
- 1 scoop protein powder
- ½ medium-sized banana (frozen)
- ½ cup frozen strawberries
- 2 tsp. ground flaxseeds or flaxseed oil

Simply add all ingredients to your blender. Blend on high for 2 minutes and enjoy!

Lunch: ***Open-Faced Tuna Sandwich and Puréed Vegetable Soup (Serves 1)***

- 4 ounces canned light tuna
- 1 tbsp. of light mayonnaise
- 2 tbsp. of diced celery
- 1 tbsp. of diced white onion
- 1 slice of whole grain bread (you can use one of your treats here by adding a second slice of bread)
- 2 slices of tomato
- 2 pieces Romaine lettuce
- 1 cup puréed vegetable soup (homemade or purchased)

Add mayonnaise to tuna and mix well in serving bowl. Chop celery and onion into small pieces and mix into tuna. Spoon tuna onto whole grain bread and top with lettuce and tomato. Enjoy with puréed vegetable soup of your choice on the side (i.e. vegetable stock, tomato soup, pea soup etc.)

Note: If purchasing a store bought soup, try to buy one with natural ingredients. Most canned soups are high in sodium. Fresh made soups in glass jars are often found in the produce section of most grocery stores.

Snack

- 1 apple or pear

Dinner: ***Scrambled Eggs, Lox and Capers (Serves 1)***

- 1 whole egg
- 1 tbsp. of diced white onion
- 4 egg whites
- 2 ounces smoked salmon, cut into thin strips (wild if possible)
- Freshly ground black pepper
- 2 tsp. capers

Whisk eggs and egg whites together. Coat a nonstick skillet with olive oil or a small amount of non-salted butter. Sautée onions and capers until tender and add egg mixture. On medium heat, gently cook eggs until they begin to take form. Use a flexible spatula to move the eggs around. Just before the eggs are set, stir in the salmon and capers.

Note: Use 1 whole egg and 4 egg whites per person. Alternatively, use egg substitute if you prefer.

Friday

Breakfast: ***Cottage Cheese Strawberry Banana Crunch (Serves 1)***

- ½ cup 1% or non-fat cottage cheese
- ½ sliced banana
- ¼ cup sliced strawberries
- ½ cup bran buds

Add cottage cheese, sliced bananas and strawberries intio serving bowl. Sprinkle ½ cup of bran buds on top and enjoy!

Lunch: ***Chicken, Apple and Walnut Salad (Serves 1)***

- 1 cooked skinless chicken breast, cubed , 4 ounces
- 1 cup celery, sliced
- 1 medium unpeeled apple, diced
- ¼ cup walnuts, crushed
- 1 tbsp. lemon juice
- ¼ cup low-fat yogurt
- ¼ cup fat-free mayonnaise
- 1 tsp. curry powder
- 1 ½ cups of lettuce or mixed greens

Place chicken cubes in a medium-sized bowl along with sliced celery, diced apple and walnuts. In a small bowl, whisk lemon juice, yogurt, mayonnaise and curry powder. Pour over chicken and toss to coat. Place on a bed of lettuce and enjoy!

Snack

- ½ cup of broccoli florets and baby carrots
- 2 tsp. of non-fat ranch dip

Dinner: ***Tuna Salad (Serves 1)***

- 1 can of light tuna in water, drained
- 2 cups mixed greens
- 1 tsp. light mayonnaise
- 2 tsp. light Italian or balsamic vinaigrette dressing
- ½ large ripe tomato, sliced

Mix tuna and mayonnaise thoroughly. If desired, you can use hand blender to mix tuna for a smoother consistency. Place tuna over top of plated mixed greens. Add sliced tomato and salad dressing.

Saturday

Breakfast: ***Omega-3 Yogurt Supreme (Serves 1)***

- ½ cup of blueberries
- 8-10 walnuts, crushed
- ½ cup of light yogurt (any flavor, naturally sweetened)

Add yogurt, blueberries and walnuts into a small bowl. Mix together and enjoy!

Lunch: ***Chicken Tomato Wrap (Serves 1)***

- ½ cup cooked chicken breast, cubed
- 2 tbsp. honey Dijon salad dressing
- 2 tbsp. mayonnaise
- ½ green pepper, diced
- 1 tomato, chopped
- 2 lettuce leaves
- 1 whole-grain or 100% whole-wheat wrap

In medium-sized bowl combine chicken, salad dressing, mayonnaise, green pepper and tomatoes, and toss. Spoon mixture onto wrap, top with lettuce leaves, fold and serve.

Snack

- 1 small yogurt

Dinner: ***BBQ Chicken Kabobs (Serves 1)***

- 1 skinless, boneless chicken breast, cubed
- 1 large green bell pepper, cut into 2-inch pieces
- 1 onion, cut into wedges
- 1 large red bell pepper, cut into 2-inch pieces
- ½ cup barbeque sauce

Preheat grill on high heat. Alternately thread the chicken, green bell pepper, onion, and red bell pepper pieces onto skewers. Lightly oil with olive oil the grill grate. Place kabobs on the grill and cook for 10 minutes, then brush with barbeque sauce for an additional 5 minutes. Take off grill and enjoy.

Sunday

Breakfast: ***Broccoli Cheesy Eggs (Serves 1)***

- 1 cup egg whites
- ½ white onion diced
- 1 ½ cups broccoli floweret's
- 1 tsp. butter
- 1 tbsp. Tex Mex seasoning
- ¼ cup soy or low-fat shredded mozzarella cheese

Melt butter in non-stick pan. Add diced onion and broccoli. Sautée until tender. Add egg and stir constantly. When mixture is ½ cooked, add salt and pepper and shredded cheese. Continue to cook until egg mixture is fully cooked.

Lunch: ***Open-Face Turkey Hummus Sandwich (Serves 1)***

- 2 tsp. hummus dip
- 1 slice whole-grain bread
- 3–4 slices deli cooked turkey
- ¼ cucumber, peeled and sliced
- 1 plum tomatoes, sliced

Spread hummus over whole-grain bread. Layer remaining ingredients on top to create open-face sandwich.

Snack: ***Homemade Popsicle (makes 6-8 Popsicles)***

- Yogurt (1 cup, any flavor, naturally sweetened)
- Orange juice (1 cup)
- ½ cup of favorite frozen fruit (i.e., mangos, blueberries)

Blend yogurt, frozen fruit and orange juice, place in Popsicle forms and freeze.

Dinner: ***Stir-Fried Tempeh and Broccoli (Serves 1)***

- 4 ounces tempeh, cut into ½-inch pieces
- 1 cup of broccoli florets
- ½ cup soy sauce
- 1 red pepper, chopped
- ½ onion, diced

Marinate tempeh in soy sauce and set aside. Heat olive oil in large nonstick skillet over high heat. Add onions and cook until tender. Add tempeh, broccoli, red pepper and sauté for 4 minutes. Add more soy sauce to taste.

Common Questions and Answers

After starting hundreds of people off on re-setting their metabolic code during the first 30 days, I've noticed that common questions tend to pop up. Since you probably have one or two of these questions on your mind, I have answered the most frequently asked questions below for your reference.

Question: My friend and I are both following the 30 days to re-setting our metabolic code. She has lost 6 pounds per week and I have only lost 2. Why is that?

Answer: Ah...the joys of weight loss! First of all, whether it is a friend, family member or co-worker, I highly recommend having a weight-loss "buddy." The more people you can be accountable to during this process, the better.

Although difficult, try not to compare your results to anyone else's. Similar to any other venture we embark on, results will differ from person to person, depending on their health history, weight-loss history and genetics. On average, people will lose two to six pounds per week in the first 30 days. If you are losing one-and-a-half to two pounds or more per week, you are definitely on the right path. Your friend may have a slightly higher metabolic rate, may be working out more or may be one of the lucky ones who drops it fast! Remember the motto, "Slow and steady wins the race." The weight-loss programs on the market that promise eight to 10 pounds of weight-loss per week are not healthy nor are they realistic or effective for long-term weight loss. The weight you lose in the first 30 days and beyond will be long lasting and manageable for life. If you are not losing two pounds or more per week, here are a few suggestions to rev it up a notch.

- For two weeks, drop your lunchtime grain to drive up glucagon secretion (a hormone that breaks down fat).
- Crank up your cardiovascular work outs to five times per week for a minimum of 30 minutes per day. Treadmill, running, elliptical machine, brisk walking, racquet sports—"get active!"

- Drink your green tea. Remember, three cups per day has been shown to promote weight loss.
- Make sure you are having a bowel movement daily. If not, please refer to the question on constipation on page 115.
- Drink a minimum of six to eight glasses of water per day. For a natural astringent effect, squeeze fresh lemon into your water.

Question: Help! I am starving—what should I do?

Answer: You should *not* be starving during the first 30 days. If you are, chances are you are not getting the proper amount of fat or protein. Proteins and fats are the two macronutrients that will fill you up for a prolonged period of time. Turn to Chapter 4 and review the proteins and fats you should be consuming daily. Here are some examples of ways to include some more fat and protein in your diet without gaining weight.

Fat

- Add flaxseed oil to your morning shake.
- Eat 8–10 almonds or walnuts.
- Eat ¼ of an avocado (added to sandwich or salad).
- Cook with olive oil.
- Eat 1 ounce of low-fat cheese.

Protein

- Add one heaping scoop of protein powder in your morning smoothie.
- Eat hard-boiled eggs for breakfast, lunch or a snack. Eggs contain both protein and fat that will fill you up, and they're easy to bring to the office!
- Have tuna, salmon, turkey, chicken or soy meats on whole-grain bread at lunch.
- Eat yogurt or cottage cheese mixed with fruits (carbohydrates) and nuts (fat).

Question: I did the 30 days, and I have been losing weight, but I still have a long way to go. How do I know when my metabolism is ready for the next step?

Answer: If you have a smaller amount of weight to lose (10–15 pounds), you have likely achieved your weight-loss goals within the first 30 days. If you are one of the rare inividuals whose metabolism is extremely sluggish (i.e., losing less than 2 pounds per week), you can safely stay on the 30 days to re-set your metabolic code for an additional month.

Question: I am experiencing terrible cravings. Is this normal?

Answer: As you will discover in more detail in Chapter 6, "Carbohydrates 101," eating the wrong foods such as refined flours and sugars will cause blood sugar fluctuations, energy dips and cravings anywhere from one-half hour to three hours following a meal or snack. One of the main objectives of the first 30 days is to balance blood sugar with food. That said, it is quite common for cravings to worsen temporarily before they subside. Keep in mind that a craving is an indication that you are hormonally imbalanced. The next time you experience a craving, take a moment to check in with what you are feeling. For example, there is a big difference between, "I would like a cookie," and "I need a cookie!" Although people continually try to fight off their cravings, in the long term, this is an exercise in futility. Cravings are an indication that you are in need of some hormonal balancing. They are also an indication that you are likely over-secreting insulin. You are not weak if you give in to them. In fact, because the craving sensation is intimately linked with blood sugar control and brain chemicals, it is very difficult not to give into them. For long-term results, it is far better to combat cravings with proper nutrition and proper blood sugar control rather than have constant feelings of deprivation.

Often times, people report they experience cravings in the mid-afternoon. We term this phenomenon the "3 p.m. slump." In essence, the time of this craving is of no coincidence. Following a lunch filled with refined flours and sugars and not enough proteins or fats, you plop back down at your desk or in your car only to experience extreme fatigue by mid-afternoon. What do you do when the feeling hits? In an attempt to bring energy up quickly, you go to the closest drive-through kiosk or coffee vendor. Unfortunately, this will keep the vicious cycle of fatigue, improper blood sugar control and weight gain happening again and again.

Remember, once your blood sugar begins to normalize and hormonal balance is achieved through food, your cravings will subside. You may enjoy eating naturally sweet fruits, whole grains, etc., but you will not "need" them. In the first week, if your cravings elevate in intensity, the following steps will help you to curb them.

- Invest in chewable vitamin C. When you do experience a sweet craving, grab two chewable capsules (usually 250–500mg each). Once your brain registers a sweet taste from the chewable vitamin C, the craving sensation will be satisfied.
- Invest in a multitude of berry herbal teas such as strawberry, blueberry, peach and orange. Make yourself a sweet cup of tea rather than indulging in a gooey treat you will only regret.
- Do not keep tempting foods in your cupboards. If cookies, cereal, granola bars or chocolate treats are around when you have a craving, chances are you will eat them.
- Keep crunchy "free foods" on hand. Eat cut-up celery, cucumbers and even baby carrots to satisfy the urge to munch.
- Read labels and watch for processed foods that contain an abundant amount of added sugar. Stick to the natural sweetness in fruit. The most optimal fruits to eat are berries such as strawberries, raspberries or blueberries because they are filled to the brim with anti-oxidants and are low on the glycemic index.
- Often times, having a sweet tooth is linked to emotional eating. For example, grabbing a sugary or starchy carbohydrate will temporarily bring energy and mood up. Yet, what goes up, must also go down. The short-lived increase in energy and mood will result in a crash soon

after, due to a state of hypoglycemia (commonly known as low blood sugar). Although difficult to do, prior to grabbing a muffin or cookie when you have a craving, stop yourself in the moment to see why you are eating. Are you hungry? Bored? Sad? Mindlessly munching? Identifying the emotion behind the food will help you to stop the behavior.

Question: I find not eating late at night very difficult. Any suggestions?

Answer: Do not despair. For most people, this is the hardest step in the book. To successfully complete this step, you need to practice the laws of creating a habit. In other words, the old adage of "practice makes perfect" is absolutely correct. Simply start by creating a pattern of repetition by not eating a minimum of three hours prior to bedtime for a minimum of one week. Within the first week, you will find that with regular practice, this new food behavior soon becomes second nature. You will also notice that the results gained from implementing this step will far outweigh the initial mental focus it will take. By not eating past 7 p.m. (or three hours before bed), your weight-loss results will occur more rapidly, and you will rise in the morning with a flatter stomach, more energy and improved digestion.

When changing any behavior, it is always best to have a replacement behavior for optimal results. In other words, when the urge to munch hits you late at night, go call a friend, fold some laundry, brush your teeth, have a glass of water or herbal tea, read a magazine or book, or take a bath. Also, late night is the time when emotional eating tends to kick in. Check in with yourself to see if you are indeed eating because you are hungry or because of feelings of loneliness or boredom. As mentioned, we all indulge in emotional eating to some degree. Once you identify the root cause, the behavior will immediately lessen and subside.

Question: What if I work shift work?

Answer: I get this question quite often from doctors, nurses, truck drivers and others whose occupations require that they work in shifts and change schedules every one or two weeks. Frankly, this is not an ideal schedule for optimal health. The body thrives on routine and the constant changing of sleep cycles can dramatically affect hormonal function. In addition, between 2 a.m. and 4 a.m. is when the body secretes a very powerful anti-cancer hormone called melatonin. Melatonin can only be secreted in complete darkness while asleep.

If you absolutely must work shift work, you need to keep a keen eye on your nutritional intake. Obviously, the "not eating past 7 p.m." rule cannot apply. The best approach is to ensure you are eating very nutrient-dense foods in the form of fresh fruits, vegetables, whole grains and protein options such as yogurt, sliced meats, nuts and seeds. In addition, it is important to stay well hydrated with water, herbal and green or white tea. Try not to over-consume during your night shift as it will leave you feeling sluggish and tired. Rather, eat light and fresh energizing foods that will keep your energy up, your weight down and will get you to the end of your shift.

Question: I was doing great until recently, and now I feel stuck! Why have I hit a plateau?

Answer: Most people hit a plateau within the first four to six weeks of losing weight. While it is unlikely that you will hit a plateau during the first few weeks of *The Last 15*, if you do, there are certain tricks of the nutritional trade that can help you break through this temporary barrier. It is also important to mention that weight loss does not always occur in a straight line. In other words, some weeks you may lose five pounds, while other weeks you may lose one or two pounds. In the first month, people often find that the weight "falls off" quickly. After approximately four to six weeks, a two-pound weight loss per week is normal and healthy.

Hitting a plateau is often an indicator that your body has adapted to your current routine and needs change. If you do hit a plateau, whether early or later on, do not panic. I have known many people to hit a one- to two-week plateau months into their weight-loss journey where they simply do not lose. Don't despair; you just need to get your metabolism "unstuck" by switching out of your adaptation mode. The following tips can help get you through this short-term situation.

- Modify and alter your exercise routine. For example, lengthen or change the type of cardiovascular workout you are doing, train with different types of weights or add different types of exercises such as squats, lunges, yoga or Pilates. The key is to get out of an adaptive rut by doing something different. Also, ensure that you are not overdoing it in terms of exercise. If you have been engaging in intense daily workouts, lighten up for a couple of weeks. The key is to focus on change to "shake your body" out of its current routine.
- Zigzag your caloric intake in order to change your schedule. In other words, if you are eating three meals and one snack per day, eat the same amount of calories but eat five to six times per day instead of three to four times per day. You want to trick your body into thinking it is doing something different.
- Temporarily boost your protein intake.
- Make sure you are well hydrated. Often times, an inability to lose weight goes hand in hand with dehydration.
- While you are in the midst of the plateau, drop alcohol. Drinking alcohol can slow down the fat-burning capabilities of the body, as the body focuses on using the alcohol as a source of fuel, rather than burning fat for energy. In addition, alcohol dehydrates the body, which, in turn, makes you hungry.
- Watch your digestion; ensure you are having one fully formed bowel movement per day.

Question: I am finding that I am constipated. What should I do?

Answer: If you are constipated in the initial week or two, I recommend adding ½ cup of bran to your morning meal to bulk up your stools. I am a huge advocate of optimal digestion. One of my most frequent sayings is, "You are only as healthy as your pipes!" By this, of course, I am referring to your entire digestive system—from mouth to anus. In other words, if you are not absorbing and excreting properly, you will not achieve your optimal health and weight. For weight loss, optimal energy and disease prevention, healthy elimination is just as important as a healthy diet.

You will likely find once you start with the ½ cup of bran cereal in the morning, you will start to eliminate properly and eventually will not need the extra fiber to bulk up stool. The vegetables, beans, fruits and whole grains you will be eating daily will be enough to promote optimal digestive health.

Question: How often should I have a bowel movement?

Answer: Although the "scoop on poop" may not be the most appetizing conversation you can have, it is of the utmost importance. Symptoms such as acne, low energy, bloating, inability to lose weight and inflammatory conditions can all be linked to faulty digestion.

A healthy digestive system will eliminate a minimum of once daily. If you are in pristine digestive health (which sadly most of us are not due to dehydration and a poor diet), you may find you have two to three fully formed bowel movements per day. What is a healthy bowel movement? Your stool should be light to medium brown, should float and ideally, should be in an "S" or "C" curve. Your stool should also leave your body without strain or discomfort.

Question: Should I go for colonics?

Answer: A colonic, also called colon hydrotherapy, is performed by a colon therapist who inserts a disposable speculum into the anus. The speculum is then connected to a long disposable plastic hose that is hooked up to a colon hydrotherapy unit. Warm water is filtered into the colon and then slowly released. The water causes contraction of the muscles of the colon which pushes the feces out through a hose to a closed water system. Colonics are touted as one of the most effective methods at eliminating fecal and bacterial build up.

While I believe that regularity is of the utmost importance to overall health, I am *not* an advocate of colonics. The digestive system is a self-regulating system, which, when in top health, absorbs and eliminates according to the body's natural rhythm. In other words, what goes in (i.e., food) should come out by itself naturally! Recent weight-loss programs are promoting colonic therapy for a number of "cures" such as cleansing and optimal weight-loss results. I have seen numerous websites promote colonics for a flatter tummy, improved energy and instant weight loss. There is no evidence to substantiate this claim, nor is it a healthy choice. I recommend you stay focused on what works in the long term —caloric and hormonal balance.

Danielle

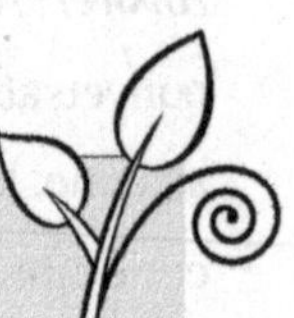

Age: 34

Height: 5 feet 6 inches

Previous weight: 154 pounds

Current weight: 137 pounds

Total weight lost: 17 pounds!

Upon first meeting Danielle, her upbeat and friendly manner was infectious. I sensed she was a winner from the start. At age 34, Danielle had recently given birth to her second child and like so many other women, had those nagging 20 extra pounds to lose.

Due to her excess weight, she reported feeling energy fluctuations and fatigue throughout the day. She also reported she was an emotional eater and often searched for sweets when stress was high. About to return to work full time, as well as juggling all of the other responsibilities of being a mom and wife, Danielle felt a considerable amount of anxiety that was contributing to her poor eating habits. It was not unusual for her to grab a handful of M&M's or banana bread when she felt stressed by family members. Although Danielle did not have a significant amount of weight to lose, getting back to her goal weight was important for her self-confidence, vitality and overall health.

After reviewing Danielle's food journal her nutritional slips, that were causing her to keep on her excess weight and drive up insulin secretion became apparent. Danielle's diet was filled with high-glycemic index choices such as refined cereals, bagels, pancakes, cookies (chocolate chip cookies were her weakness), pasta, chocolate and muffins. She also reported having intense food cravings and often snacking between 9 and 10 p.m. She felt a little nervous at the thought of giving up all her goodies such as banana bread, but she knew she needed a health boost. At 5 feet 6 inches, Danielle first weighed in at 154 pounds with a waist circumference of 36 inches.

After our initial meeting, I assured Danielle that she would not be giving up delicious eating. In fact, she would still be able to have some sweet treats throughout the week, all the while losing weight. Initially, I recommended that Danielle cut out all refined flour and sugar products from her diet and boost her green tea and water intake. Danielle started each day with a creamy protein shake, learned to seek out proteins at each and every meal and was enjoying low-glycemic index carbohydrates such as whole-grain bread, fruits, vegetables and the occasional baked good. She also started an exercise routine by walking and kickboxing two times per week. After a short time, Danielle reported how easy and attainable her new way of eating was. Once she understood the hormonal balance approach, when she did fall off the health wagon during times of stress, she knew how to climb back on. She also paid more attention to her emotional triggers and instead of soothing herself with food, she made wiser choices such as being with her children, having green tea, exercising or snacking on low-glycemic fruits and vegetables. Her intense sweet cravings soon started to subside as her baby weight started to melt off leaving her with the extra energy she needed to keep up with her baby daughter and her toddler son.

I saw Danielle a couple of months ago and she looked fantastic—svelte, fit and very energetic. I am proud to say, she has reached her goal weight of 135 pounds and is down nearly 10 inches overall! I am very impressed by this busy working mom for achieving and sticking to her goal. Her connection with food was both physical (hormonal imbalance) and emotional. With careful focus and dedication, she turned her health around in under three months! Trust me, if she could carve out the time for health and wellness, we all can.

Danielle did not have to dramatically change her hectic schedule or the time she spent with her children. That was simply not a realistic change for her. She did, however, sharpen her focus on her food choices by eliminating processed goods from the diet and replacing them with lean proteins, essential fats and low-glycemic index carbohydrates. Danielle also strictly followed the 30 days to re-setting her metabolic code, which facilitated the initial spark that caused all the weight to melt away.

part 2

The Rest of Your Life!

Once you have hit your goal weight, you are ready for Part 2—the rest of your life! This section will provide you with all you need to know about hormonal balance and the three basic macronutrients; 1) carbohydrates, 2) proteins, and 3) fats. In addition, I will lay out the steps necessary to create permanent health and to maintain your weight loss. From the top 10 disease-preventing foods to reading labels and guiltless snacking—it is all included in Part 2. I assure you, people who are nutritional students for life are always the ones who are the healthiest and have the easiest time maintaining a lean body weight.

Keep in mind we are all in a constant dance with food. There will be many occasions such as weddings, Christmas, Thanksgiving, and other special occasions and holidays where we tend to eat a little too much at the dessert table or have one too many alcoholic beverages. This type of "cheating" is simply part of life and part of the fun of treating yourself once in a while. That said, the food options outlined in the recipe section in the back of the book and in Part 2 are so delicious and satisfying that you will not experience salt or sugar cravings that lead to unhealthy food choices.

As in other areas of life such as your finances, career and relationships, knowledge is power. In other words, once you have the proper nutritional background and understanding, you will be able to find hormonal and caloric balance at any time, making your weight-loss struggles a thing of the past.

6

Carbohydrates 101

"The higher your energy level, the more efficient your body. The more efficient your body, the better you feel and the more you will use your talent to produce outstanding results."

Anthony Robbins,
American author, speaker, peak performance expert and consultant

When it comes to weight loss and the foods we love, carbohydrates top the chart. Think about it. When you crave a food, do you crave an egg? A piece of celery? Of course not! People typically crave a sugary or starchy carbohydrate such as a slice of banana bread or a cookie. Yet, due to the low-carbohydrate diet craze that was recently on an upswing, North American weight-loss seekers everywhere were dropping this precious macronutrient in an attempt to lose weight. I literally had clients report that when going "hard core" low carbohydrate, they would drive through a local fast food restaurant, order a hamburger, discard the bun and eat only the beef patty in an attempt to lose weight fast. Did it work? It did indeed, but only temporarily and in a very unhealthy manner. Most did not sustain the short-term weight loss results and ended up feeling fatigued and moody. They also had more inflammation such as achy joints and suffered from constipation. As we have seen, it is far worse for your health to gain and lose weight repetitively. That is why becoming a nutritional student and keeping it off for good (with the occasional indulgence here and there!) is far healthier.

The core message of this chapter focuses on one theme: when it comes to weight loss and hormonal balance, all carbohydrates are *not* created equal. Once you can decipher the good from the bad, you will be able to incorporate all types of carbohydrates into your daily diet without gaining weight.

What Are Carbohydrates?

Carbohydrates are the sugars and starches found in breads, cereals, fruits, vegetables and beans. When eaten, carbohydrates are broken down into a simple sugar called glucose which is the key form of energy or fuel for the body. When the glucose is not needed for immediate energy, it is stored in the liver and muscles as glycogen. Glycogen can be broken down by the body at any time and used for fuel when excess glucose is not available. The liver and muscles only have limited storage space and once full, the excess glucose from eating too many grams of carbohydrates will be stored as fat. This is a key point: eating too many carbohydrate-dense, high-glycemic index carbohydrates equals fat!

So why all the fuss about low-carbohydrate diets for optimal weight-loss results? One of the key determinants of how good a carbohydrate is partially depends on the speed of entry of a carbohydrate into the bloodstream. Carbohydrates that enter the bloodstream at a rushing speed cause a greater secretion of the pancreatic hormone insulin. Excess insulin secretion can ultimately lead to weight gain (especially around the abdominal region), type 2 diabetes and heart disease. A scale that has been at the forefront of measuring the speed of entry of carbohydrates into the bloodstream is called the glycemic index. For ranking purposes, the glycemic index is divided into three categories; low, medium and high. Food is classified from a scale of 0 to 100 depending on its effect on blood sugar levels. On the glycemic scale, the highest measurement is for glucose, which has a ranking of 100. Individual foods with a high-glycemic index rating release glucose into the bloodstream quickly, thereby causing blood sugar levels to rise rapidly. Foods that are rated lower on the glycemic index have slower rate of entry into the blood stream and therefore lower insulin response. These foods release glucose more steadily over several hours, helping to keep blood sugar levels relatively balanced. The categories of the glycemic index are summarized below.

Low (up to 55)
Medium (56–70)
High (over 70)

How Many Carbohydrates?

Although the glycemic index (GI) is a very helpful tool in determining what and how you eat, it should not be the only criteria. The total amount of carbohydrates, the amount and type of fat, and the fiber and salt content are also important dietary considerations. That said, when selecting carbohydrates, sticking to low- to medium-glycemic index carbohydrates for weight loss is recommended. In fact, more than 17 studies confirm that eating foods with a low-GI value keeps you satisfied longer than eating high-GI foods.

For weight-loss and weight maintenance (and depending on activity level, intensity and number of workouts per week) your carbohydrate intake should be approximately 80 to 140 grams per day. For individuals who are highly active, this number may increase slightly. For others who are fairly inactive, overweight or insulin-resistant, a lower carbohydrate diet is best. While some food guides recommend eating 50 to 60% of total calories from carbohydrate intake, I think this is far too high and not necessary. In addition, it is also likely one of the reasons we are seeing a major upswing in disease processes such as type 2 diabetes and obesity. For weight loss and optimal health, approximately 40% of all the calories you eat should be derived from carbohydrates. Science confirms this. Research has clearly shown that diets filled with low-glycemic index carbohydrates (30 to 40% of the daily diet), lean proteins (30%) and essential fats (25 to 30%) are optimal for weight management and blood sugar control.

Below are examples of the number of grams of carbohydrates in a variety of foods. Combining this information with the selection of low- to medium-GI foods will keep your blood sugar in check, your hormones balanced and your weight down. Now that you have completed your 30-day metabolic boost, your typical carbohydrate intake per day should consist of:

- 2–4 servings of grains
- 5–8 servings of vegetables
- 2–3 servings of fruit

Average serving sizes are outlined on the following page:

Bread, Cereal, Rice, Pasta, Beans and Starchy Vegetables: 15 g of Carbohydrate per Serving

1 slice bread (1 oz)

¼ bagel

¾ cup dry cereal

½ cup cooked cereal

⅓ cup cooked rice or pasta

½ cup cooked dry beans, lentils, peas, or corn

¼ large baked potato

Vegetables: 5 g of Carbohydrate per Serving

1 cup of raw leafy vegetables

½ cup other vegetables, cooked or raw

¾ cup vegetable juice

Fruits: 15 g of Carbohydrate per Serving

1 medium apple, banana or orange

½ cup chopped, cooked or canned fruit

½ cup fruit juice

¼ cup dried fruit

After eating, the time it takes for the body to convert carbohydrates and release glucose into the bloodstream varies, depending on the type of carbohydrate. Some carbohydrate-rich foods such as refined flour and sugars cause the blood glucose level to rise rapidly, while others have a more gradual effect. In order to understand how different carbohydrates are processed in the body, let us examine two scenarios.

Scenario 1: Fast-Car, High-GI Carbohydrates

High-GI carbohydrates are typically made from refined flours and sugars. In the processing of these items, the foods have been stripped of their precious fiber content, leaving behind a white fluffy flour or sugar to make products such as white bread, white pasta, muffins, cookies, cakes, cereals, granola bars, candy and soda pop. The popularization of stripping grains and adding sugars to a myriad of products is relatively new in the food industry (with a surge in the past 50 years) and is doing a great disservice to the healthcare system in North America. Without even being aware, consumers are eating food items that are loaded with the wrong type of flour and are consuming an enormous amount of added sugar.

Fiber is one of the key ingredients that slows down the entry of a carbohydrate into the bloodstream. When fiber is stripped from a whole grain or sugar cane and a white crystalline powder is left to make baked goods or other processed goodies, the brakes are eliminated and the carbohydrate zooms into the bloodstream at a very fast speed—like a fast car. When this occurs, the pancreas is alerted to the situation and secretes the hormone insulin in response. Of insulin's many roles, one is to transport excess blood sugar into the cells for use.

Now, if this situation happens once or twice, it is really no big deal and the body handles it. However, if you routinely eat the wrong type of bread, pasta, highly sugared or high-glycemic index carbohydrates on a daily basis, your blood sugar roller coasters and you will be thrown out of hormonal balance. For example, when blood sugar (glucose) is elevated at a dramatic rate day in and day out by eating high-glycemic foods, the body sends out a response to deal with the high levels of blood glucose. This elevated state of blood sugar is called *hyperglycemia*. Keep in mind that the body's main job is to maintain a state of balance called homeostasis. If the body thinks something is out of whack such as blood sugar that is too high, it triggers a response to deal with the situation. For high blood sugar, the response is to trigger the pancreas to secrete more and more insulin.

So how does this result in weight gain? If an individual continually eats high-GI carbohydrates, the pancreas starts to chug out more and more insulin to deal with the excess of blood sugar (glucose). The problem occurs on three fronts:

1. The individual who was once hyperglycemic (high blood sugar) is now hypoglycemic (low blood sugar). This occurs due to the excess of insulin secreted. Hypoglycemic individuals commonly experience symptoms such as fatigue, fogginess and food cravings. Remember, you do not normally crave a protein, fruit or veggie; you crave something sweet or starchy. When you reach for the closest sugary treat or snack one to three hours after eating a high-glycemic index food, you continue the vicious cycle that bounces around blood sugar, energy levels and intensifies cravings for the wrong foods. Think about this situation the next time you feel sleepy or groggy after eating a meal. Instead of accepting that you experience a window of fatigue day in and day out, the "3 p.m. slump," look at your previous meal or snack. Was your lunch or snack heavy on fast-car carbohydrates?
2. Insulin is a fat-storage hormone. Thus, when excess insulin is secreted, it results in the excess storage of fat! Until excess insulin is under control, losing weight and maintaining hormonal balance is next to impossible. This is one of the key areas the first 30 days focuses on. Once your insulin secretion is normalized with proper foods such as lean protein, high-fiber options and essential fats, the pounds will melt away and your energy will surge.
3. Excess insulin secretion can result in various ill health effects such as heart disease and type 2 diabetes. With heart disease the number one killer in North America and type 2 diabetes following closely behind, hormonal balance through food is of the utmost importance.

High-GI Foods to Avoid or Minimize

White bread

White rolls

Baguette

Bagel

Dried dates

Instant mashed potatoes
Baked white potato
Parsnips
Rutabaga
Instant rice
Many cereals (Corn Flakes, Rice Krispies, Cheerios, puffed wheat, shredded wheat)
Soda crackers
Jellybeans
French fries
Pretzels
Corn chips
Rice cakes
Doughnuts
Waffles

What about Bread?

When I travel to speak on weight loss and health, I receive many questions on the hot nutritional topics. The question about bread is one that always pops up. I often see skeptical faces when I mention that eating the right type of bread is totally acceptable for weight loss and weight maintenance. In fact, I can always pinpoint the hard-core low-carb dieters in the crowd. They are the ones that appear confused with a scrunched up look on their face, as if to say, "Do you mean that bread is back in?" In truth, bread was never "out." However, eating the right type of bread and the proper amount is critical to weight-loss success. Remember, the key is to select low- to medium-GI carbohydrates in a suitable portion size.

If you visit your local grocery store bakery or bread section, you will find there is enormous variety: white bread to seven grain, whole grain, whole wheat, rye, sprouted and omega-3 enriched. You name it; you can find it. With all this selection, it is important to keep in mind that you need to drastically minimize bread made from white, refined and bleached flour. This bread is a high-GI carbohydrate that will promote the oversecretion of insulin. In fact, your body has no idea if it is eating a piece of white refined bread or a drinking a can of pop. All the body knows is that it is getting high-GI carbohydrates and that it better respond by pumping out insulin. Consider some of the following GI ratings for bread made of refined, white flour bread.

- White French baguette: 90 (high)
- White rolls: 73 (high)
- White piece of bread: 70 (high)

In an attempt to avoid white bread and refined flours, many people seek out whole wheat. It seems like that should make sense, doesn't it? This bread sounds like it is healthy with the word "whole" in front of the name. It even looks healthier with its medium to dark brown hue. However, not all whole-wheat bread is created equal. In fact, in Canada, it is legal to advertise any food product as "whole wheat" with up to 70% of the germ removed (a precious part of the grain that contains nutrient value), whereas in the United States whole-wheat flour contains all three parts of the grain, making it a whole-grain product.

Whole-grain bread has been receiving a lot of attention for its health benefits. It is made from the entire grain kernel—the bran, the germ and the endosperm. Refined grains only contain the endosperm. Research now shows that the bran contains beneficial fiber, B vitamins and trace minerals, while the germ contains anti-oxidants, vitamin E and B vitamins as well. The nutritional advantages of eating the entire grain has been linked with numerous health benefits such as lowering the incidence of some forms of cancer, digestive diseases, coronary heart disease, diabetes and even obesity. In fact, a variety of studies have shown eating high-fiber whole grains to be quite beneficial for long-term weight-loss success.

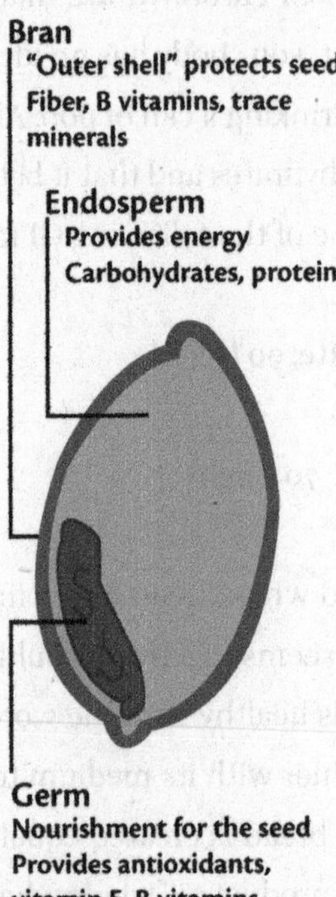

The key to making sure you are selecting high-quality, healthy bread is to become a savvy label reader. Simply follow the steps below to make sure you are selecting properly.

Dr. Joey's Bread Test

- When selecting bread, check the ingredients list and look for the words 100% "whole wheat" or "whole grain" before the name of the grain. Terms such as "wheat flour" generally indicates it is not derived from the entire grain and therefore is not a whole-grain product.
- Whole grain breads typically contain more fiber. Look for a minimum of 2 grams of fiber for every slice of bread.
- Do not be fooled by the words, "fortified with." Fortification typically occurs with refined grains. Precious nutrients that have been stripped away during the refining process are added back in. Manufacturers

are sometimes required by law to fortify refined grain products to make up for the loss of vitamins and minerals.

- If there is a phone number on the packaging, contact the company to see if they have the GI rating of the bread in question.
- When picking up the bread, it should actually feel slightly heavier due to the higher fiber content. You will not be able to roll this bread into a small ball like you can with white bread. This bread does not "melt in your mouth" and has to be chewed well.
- After you eat the bread, notice if you feel tired soon after. Food items that are higher on the glycemic index cause your blood sugar to fluctuate and often leave you in a hypoglycemic (low blood sugar) and fatigued state. This is also the time that cravings for starch or sugar usually kick in.
- Look at the ingredients list rather than the color of the bread to select whole-grain foods.

Look for Omega-3 bread options. Omega-3 is an essential fat necessary for optimal health that can only be obtained by the diet. See Chapter 8 for more details on these fats.

- Eat sprouted grain. Sprouted grain bread is "live" bread made with sprouted whole kernel grains that are mashed into dough. The benefits of the sprouting process result in a bread that is rich in minerals, vitamins, active enzymes and lignans (plant estrogens that have been shown to offer protection against heart disease and a variety of cancers). In addition, the sprouting process reduces almost all the starches (starches = carbohydrates) in the grain, thereby lowering the glycemic index of the bread. For more information on whole-grain and sprouted breads, please refer to the recommended product section at the back of the book.

I recommend eating two to four slices of whole-grain bread per day once you are past the 30 days to re-setting your metabolic code. If you wish to continue losing weight at a more rapid level, limit your bread intake to two slices per day. For those who require a wheat-free or gluten-free diet, please refer to Appendix 6.1 for information on appropriate grains.

What about Pasta?

With pasta, it is also best to stick to whole-grain options such as 100% whole-wheat pasta (i.e., spaghetti, rotini or linguine), or kamut or spelt pasta—ancient grains that are relatives of wheat. If you cannot find these pastas in your local grocery stores, most health food stores will carry them.

Due to the protein structure of pasta dough, most pasta will have a GI rating of approximately 30 to 60. In order to eat pasta without gaining weight:

- Cook your pasta el dente (undercook by 2 to 3 minutes). By doing so, you will maintain the fiber and thereby lower the GI.
- Try to have your pasta with a protein source (chicken, seafood, soy) and a lot of colorful vegetables.
- Do not over-consume pasta. ½ cup to 1 cup a couple times per week is plenty.
- Replace high-fat cheese sauces or creams with low-fat cheese, non-fat yogurt, tofu or low-fat milk.
- Enjoy some tomato sauce on your pasta! Cooked tomatoes contain a powerful anti-cancer plant chemical called lycopene. Lycopene has shown to offer powerful protection against prostate cancer. The absorption of lycopene in tomatoes is increased in the presence of fat. Therefore, add olive oil to your tomato sauce to increase absorption.
- Add flavor with garlic, onions, herbs and spices.
- Minimize brown rice pasta in the diet as it has the highest GI rating of all pastas—92.

Although certain pastas have a lower GI rating, they are still very carbohydrate-dense and should be eaten on a limited basis. The GI ratings and the grams of carbohydrates in a variety of pastas are summarized in the following table.

Glycemic Index of Various Pastas

Food	GI Value
Fettuccini (egg)	32
Spaghetti, whole wheat	37
Star Pastina	38
Spaghetti, white	38
Spiral Pasta	43
Capellini	45
Linguine	46
Macaroni	47
Rice vermicelli	58

Carbohydrate Grams in Pasta

Pasta (serving size, 1 cup cooked)	Carbs (g)
Macaroni, whole wheat	37g
Spaghetti, whole wheat	37g
Macaroni	40g
Spaghetti	40g
Lasagna, Verdi	44g
Tagliatelle	44g

For a delicious dinner option that has the perfect amount of pasta, refer to the Broccoli flower pasta (page 243) and the Squashed spaghetti (page 244) recipes.

What about Cereal?

I have often encountered many individuals who eat fairly well until approximately 6 or 7 p.m., and then they lose it—with cereal! I have actually witnessed several people who packed on extra pounds very quickly by eating high-GI cereal. Another common scenario is the individual who consumes a large bowl of sugary cereal as his morning meal and, due to blood sugar fluctuations, feels tired, moody and has cravings taunting him to eat the wrong food by 10 a.m.! Even worse, his "sugar high" in the morning rings the insulin bell and promotes excess fat storage.

It is evident that cereal is big business in North America. Part of the reason why cereal is so popular is the "convenience factor." Cereal is quick and easy to grab when you are hungry or in a rush. However, if you select the wrong one, it can be a nutritional disaster! Consider some of the cereal facts in the United States.

- Americans buy 2.7 billion packages of breakfast cereal each year. If laid end to end, the empty cereal boxes from one year's consumption would stretch to the moon and back.
- The cereal industry uses 816 million pounds of sugar per year, enough to coat each and every American with more than three pounds of sugar. The cereal with the highest amount of sugar per serving is Smacks, which is 53% sugar.
- Americans consume about 10 pounds, or 160 bowls of cereal, per person each year.
- 49% of Americans start each morning with a bowl of cereal.
- In terms of dollar value, breakfast cereals are the third most popular product sold at supermarkets, after carbonated beverages and milk. Cigarettes are the fourth most popular item followed by fresh bread and rolls.
- In 1993, more than 1.3 million advertisements for cereal aired on American television, or more than 25 hours of cereal advertising per day, at a cost of $762 million for air time. Only auto manufacturers spend more money on television advertising than the makers of breakfast cereal.

Similar to becoming label savvy when selecting bread, it is also important to be armed with nutritional information when selecting cereal. To help decide if a certain box of cereal merits a place in your kitchen pantry, consider the following cereal tips before buying.

- Purchase cereals that list the top ingredients as whole grains, whole wheat or wheat bran, not just wheat.

- Consider All-Bran. Although the germ and the endosperm are not part of the bran, it is incredibly high in fiber, loaded with nutrition and is low on the GI at 38.
- The protein content should be a minimum of 3 grams per serving. There are now several whole-grain cereals available that are higher in fiber and protein such as Kashi cereal.
- Ensure the carbohydrate-to-sugar ratio is no less than four to one. For example, if the "Total Carbohydrate" line reads 24 grams, the sugars should have a value of 6 grams or less. This means that most of the carbohydrates from the cereal are derived from grains and fiber, not sugar. However, if a cereal with 28 grams of total carbohydrate has 15 grams of sugar, the cereal in question has a far too high sugar content.
- Try to maintain the "5 in 5" rule of cereal eating. Less that 5 grams of sugar per serving, with at least 5 grams of fiber per serving.
- Use low-fat milk or soy milk on your cereal.
- Add sweetness to your morning cereal with blueberries, strawberries, sliced apples or pears.
- Do not consume cereals that contain hydrogenated oils, dyes or artificial colors or chemical preservatives.
- Ignore catchy claims on the front of cereal boxes. Go straight to the nutrition facts label for the information you need.

In addition to cereal, be careful of high-glycemic and sugar-laden breakfast options such as muffins, instant oatmeal, bagels and breakfast bars. These items will leave you feeling sluggish, hungry and craving more by approximately 10 a.m. and will pack on extra weight.

GI Breakfast Rating Chart

Low GI	Medium GI	High GI
Low fat yogurt = 15	Bran muffin = 60	Cheerios = 74
Grapefruit = 25	Instant oatmeal = 66	Cornflakes = 92
All bran cereal = 38	Whole wheat bread = 69	Rice Crispies = 82
Slow-cooking oatmeal = 49	Quick cooking oats = 65	Plain white baguette = 95

What about Rice?

Wild rice, instant white rice and sticky rice have the highest glycemic index rating and cause the most dramatic fluctuations in blood sugar. The determining factor is the ratio of amylose (the inner portion of a starch granule) to amylopectin (the outer portion of a starch granule). Rice with the lowest amount of amylose (sticky rice), has the highest GI rating. Conversely, long grain rice has the highest amylose rating and therefore, the lowest GI rating.

GI Ratings for Rice

Rice	GI rating
Converted white	38
Long grain white	44
Brown	55
Basmati	58
Short grain, white	64
Instant white	87
Wild rice	87
Glutinous, sticky rice	96

In addition to the GI rating, it is also important to watch your carbohydrate count. On average, it is best to eat less dense carbohydrates, as a majority of your carbohydrate intake. In other words, ½ cup of long grain brown rice is ideal one to two times per week.

Scenario 2: Slow-Car, Low- to Medium-Gl Carbohydrates

Unlike high-GI carbohydrates that zoom into the blood stream and cause dramatic blood sugar fluctuations, insulin secretion and weight gain, low- to medium-GI carbohydrates enter the bloodstream at a slower rate. This is because these nutrient-dense foods contain an abundant amount of fiber which acts as brakes and slows down the speed of entry. For example, if you eat high-quality carbohydrates such as broccoli, spinach, whole-grain bread, chickpeas or berries, these foods trickle into the bloodstream at a speed that does not trigger the "bell" in the pancreas to start over-secreting insulin. Instead, your body secretes an appropriate amount of insulin to deal with the blood sugar (glucose) available. With the appropriate amount of blood sugar secreted, episodes of hyperglycemia (high blood sugar) or hypoglycemia (low blood sugar) do not occur. The result? Sustained energy, hormonal balance, weight loss and a diet filled with disease-preventing foods.

Impact of High- vs. Low- to Medium-GI Foods

High GI Foods:

Raise blood sugar (hyperglycemia) ▶ insulin surge ▶ fat storage and energy fluctuations

---

Low- to Medium-GI Foods:

Normal insulin secretion ▶ weight maintenance or weight loss and sustained energy levels

---

Here are some examples of the glycemic index of various food groups.

Fruits

Food	GI Value		
Cherries	22	Pear, canned	43
Grapefruit	25	Grapes	46
Prunes	29	Papaya	56
Apricots, dried	30	Banana	52
Apple	38	Kiwi	58
Peach, canned in juice	38	Fruit cocktail	55
Pear, fresh	38	Mango	51
Plum, fresh	39	Apricots, fresh	57
Strawberries, fresh	40	Figs, dried	61
Orange, navel	42	Apricots, canned	64
Peach, fresh	42	Raisins	56
		Cantaloupe	65

Pineapple, fresh	66
Watermelon	72
Dates	103

Vegetables

Food	GI Value
Broccoli	10
Cabbage	10
Lettuce	10
Mushrooms	10
Onions	10
Red peppers	10
Carrots	49
Green peas	48
Corn, fresh	60
Beets	64
Pumpkin	75
Parsnips	97

Potatoes (Fresh)

Food	GI Value
Yam	37
Sweet	44
New	57
White skinned mashed	70
French fries	75
Instant mashed	86
Red skinned, boiled	88
Baked	85

Beans and Peas

Food	GI Value
Chana dal	8
Chickpeas, dried	28
Kidney beans, dried	28
Lentils	29
Lima beans (frozen)	32
Yellow split Peas	32
Chickpeas, canned	42
Black-eyed peas, canned	42
Baked beans	48
Kidney beans, canned	52

Breads

Food	GI Value
Pumpernickel	41
Sourdough	53
Stone ground whole wheat	53
Stonemill sprouted grains—3 grain head	55
Pita, whole wheat	57
Whole meal rye	58
Whole wheat	77
Taco shell	68
Bagel	72
White	70
Kaiser roll	73
Bread stuffing	74
French baguette	95

Crackers

Food	GI Value
Ryvita crispbread	69
Stoned wheat Thins	67
Melba toast	70
Kavli Crispbread	71
Soda Crackers	74
Graham Crackers	74
Water Crackers	78
Rice cakes	82
Rice crackers	91

Snack foods

Food	GI Value
Hummus	6
Peanuts	14
Walnuts	15
Cashews	22
FIFTY 50 Milk Chocolate Bar	30
M&M Peanut Candies	33
Milk Chocolate	43
Potato chips	57
Kudos Bar	62
Corn Chips	63
Popcorn	72
Jelly Beans	78
Pretzels	83

Keep in mind that the GI is not an indicator of health. It is merely a tool that has been designed to measure the speed of entry of a carbohydrate into the bloodstream. If understood and incorporated with other healthy eating principles, it can indeed have a dramatic and positive long-term weight-loss effect. The goal is to minimize high-GI refined flour and sugar products that tend to cause the body to over-secrete insulin and knock you out of hormonal balance.

In addition to fiber, other elements that can lower the GI of a food are fat and protein. This is one of the reasons why peanut M&M's have such a low-GI rating at 33. It is not because they are a healthy food choice. That would have been front page news by now, my friends—"Candy for weight loss!" It is because they are loaded with fat in the peanut. This is also why walnuts and cashews have such a low GI. As you will see in Chapter 8, "Fats 101," you can certainly eat fats and lose weight, but you need to know how.

What Is the Glycemic Load?

While the glycemic index is a very effective tool at measuring the speed of entry of a carbohydrate into the blood stream, it takes into account other factors that may impact speed of entry such as fat, fiber and protein. An additional tool called the glycemic load (GL) is also effective and may even be more accurate at measuring glucose entry and insulin response. The glycemic load (GL) differs from the glycemic index because it takes the amount of carbohydrates per serving into account. The calculation of the GL is the glycemic index divided by 100 and multiplied by its available carbohydrate content.

In order to understand the usefulness of the glycemic load, let's take the example of watermelon. Watermelon has a high glycemic index rating of 72. However, the glycemic load of watermelon is quit low. A 100 gram slice of watermelon with a GI of 72 and a carbohydrate content of 5 grams (watermelon contains a lot of water) would make the calculation 72/100 x 5 = 3.6. This is quite a low glycemic load rating. Both the glycemic index and glycemic load are excellent tools for measuring insulin and blood sugar response. As a general rule all foods that are low on the glycemic index tend to be low on the glycemic load (with the exception of cerain pastas due to their higher amount of carbohydrate grams). However, not all foods with a high glycemic index rating will have a high glycemic load rating (i.e. watermelon). It depends on the carbohydrate grams in the food product.

Value	Glycemic Index (GI)	Glycemic Load (GL)
High	Over 70	20
Medium	56-70	11-19
Low	Up to 55	10 or less

If you are feeling confused with the GI and GL ratings, simply keep the following carbohydrate rules in mind to keep you on track;

- Increase the consumption of whole grains, nuts, legumes, fruits and nonstarchy vegetables.
- Decrease the consumption of starchy high-glycemic index foods like potatoes, white rice and white bread.

- Decrease the consumption of sugary foods like cookies, cakes, candy and soft-drinks.

Examples of the GI and GL ratings of various food include:

Food	Glycemic Index (Glucose =100)	Serving size	Carbohydrate per serving (g)	Glycemic Load per serving
Dates, dried	103	2 oz	40	42
Cornflakes	81	1 cup	26	21
Jelly Beans	78	1 oz	28	22
Puffed rice cakes	78	3 cakes	21	17
Russet potato (baked)	76	1 medium	30	23
Doughnut	76	1 medium	23	17
Soda crackers	74	4 crackers	17	12
White bread	73	1 large slice	14	10
Table sugar (sucrose)	68	2 tsp	10	7
Pancake	67	6" diameter	58	39
White rice (boiled)	64	1 cup	36	23
Brown rice (boiled)	55	1 cup	33	18
Spaghetti, white; boiled 10-15 min	44	1 cup	40	18
Spaghetti, white; boiled 5 min	38	1 cup	40	15
Spaghetti, whole wheat; boiled	37	1 cup	37	14
Rye, pumpernickel bread	41	1 large slice	12	5
Oranges, raw	42	1 medium	11	5
Pears, raw	38	1 medium	11	4
Apples, raw	38	1 medium	15	6
All-Bran™ cereal	38	1 cup	23	9
Skim milk	32	8 fl oz	13	4
Lentils, dried; boiled	29	1 cup	18	5
Kidney beans, dried; boiled	28	1 cup	25	7

continued

Food	Glycemic Index (Glucose =100)	Serving size	Carbohydrate per serving (g)	Glycemic Load per serving
Pearled barley; boiled	25	1 cup	42	11
Cashew nuts	22	1 oz	9	2
Peanuts	14	1 oz	6	1

What Are Anti-Oxidants?

Nature is very wise and often packages healthy foods with numerous properties. When it comes to fruits and vegetables, beans and peas, most have a low-GI rating, and offer an abundant amount of mineral, vitamin and anti-oxidant capacity.

Anti-oxidants are molecules found in foods that can slow or prevent the oxidation of other chemicals that cause free radical damage. Simply put, free radical damage is cellular damage that can be caused by a number of underlying reasons such as stress, smoking, lack of exercise, food chemicals, poor air and/or water, and excess weight. Free radical damage triggers a number of reactions such as inflammation, poor digestion, low energy and suppressed immune system response. Luckily, by eating high anti-oxidant foods, you can tip the scales back, restore health and help prevent disease. In fact, research indicates that a variety of anti-oxidants have disease-preventing benefits for cancer, heart disease and inflammatory conditions such as arthritis.

In food science, the oxygen radical absorbance capacity (ORAC) has become the current industry standard for assessing the anti-oxidant capacity in whole foods and juices. In 2004, *The Journal of Agricultural and Food Chemistry* reported a new research study that focused on the anti-oxidant capacities of over 100 common foods. This study is the most comprehensive analysis of anti-oxidants in foods to date.

Best Sources of Food Antioxidants: Top 20 Fruits, Vegetables and Nuts

Rank Food	Item	Serving Size	Total antioxidant capacity per serving size
1	Small red beans (dried)	1/2 cup	13727
2	Wild blueberries	1 cup	13427
3	Red kidney beans (dried)	½ cup	13259
4	Pinto beans	½ cup	11864
5	Blueberries (cultivated)	1 cup	9019
6	Cranberries	1 cup (whole)	8983
7	Artichokes (cooked)	1 cup (hearts)	7904
8	Blackberries	1 cup	7701
9	Prunes	½ cup	7291
10	Raspberries	1 cup	6058
11	Strawberries	1 cup	5938
12	Red Delicious apples	1	5900
13	Granny Smith apples	1	5381
14	Pecans	1 ounce	5095
15	Sweet cherries	1 cup	4873
16	Black plums	1	4844
17	Russet potatoes (cooked)	1	4649
18	Black beans (dried)	½ cup	4181
19	Plums	1	4118
20	Gala apples	1	3903

Other high anti-oxidant foods include oranges, avocados, pears, broccoli, walnuts, asparagus, grapefruit and red grapes. Although spices are generally consumed in small amounts, ground cloves, ground cinnamon and oregano are among the highest anti-oxidant spices. Do you want more good news? Red wine, dark chocolate, and green and white tea have also been shown to have anti-oxidant properties!

The Bottom Line on Carbohydrates

- Carbohydrates are one of three macronutrients that are necessary in the daily diet.
- Carbohydrates are the body's main source of fuel.
- On average, an active adult should consume approximately 80 to 140 grams of carbohydrates per day. A higher intake may be necessary if an individual's activity level is high.
- A diet focused on hormonal balance and weight loss and health maintenance should consist of 80 to 90% of all carbohydrates derived from low- to medium-glycemic index choices. The lower the GI rating, the better. These selections should come from high-quality choices such as whole grains, vegetables, fruits and beans.
- The body will tend to over-secrete insulin in response to high-GI carbohydrates, which will, in turn, result in weight gain, energy fluctuation, cravings and may even lead to type 2 diabetes.
- Insulin control through diet and exercise is one of the major keys to long-term weight-loss success.

Kristine

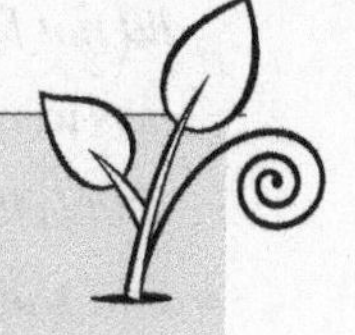

Age: 39

Height: 5 feet 3 inches

Previous Weight: 171 pounds

Current Weight: 140 pounds

Total weight lost: 31 pounds

Total lost off hips, waist and chest: 16.5 inches!

Kristine is an upbeat and friendly mother of two who had a busy schedule which included early work hours and making dinner each night for her family. At our first meeting, it was obvious that Kristine was eager to find a weight-loss program that worked. She described herself as a "chronic dieter" who had been on a very popular weight-loss program (that will remain nameless) five times! She had gained most of her weight with both pregnancies (50 pounds) and did not lose it after the pregnancy with her second child. In addition to her strong family history of heart disease and type 2 diabetes, her excess weight was also causing her to feel sluggish, irritable and lacking in confidence.

Upon first reviewing Kristine's food journal, it was obvious that she needed to make some major changes. For starters, she was drinking three to five coffees per day, two diet colas and very little water. This habit was causing her digestive system to suffer and her energy to be extremely low. She also reported eating a late night snack of cereal or cookies. If she skipped a meal, she became edgy and shaky and extremely fatigued throughout the day. Kristine's diet was also filled with high-GI carbohydrates such as muffins, cinnamon buns and cookies. By eating these on a regular basis, she was causing her blood sugar levels to fluctuate wildly, storing excess fat and increasing her risk for type 2 diabetes.

After implementing the first 30 days of The Last 15, Kristine started to lose weight; she was completely dedicated and on track. She reported enjoying her morning breakfast of a protein shake, had her grain and protein at lunch, an afternoon snack and a delicious grain-free dinner. She did not feel hungry and her nagging cravings soon subsided. Once the 30 days were over, Kristine still continued to lose weight, even with occasional "small cheats" here and there. She also decided to stay on the 30 days plan until she hit her goal weight (which she did in just over three months). Krisitine felt completely satiatied and satisfied with what she was eating and did not experience feelings of deprivation. She increased her workouts, doing Karate two to three times per week and also walking 30 minutes daily. Kristine also supplemented with a high-quality fish oil to ensure she was getting enough essential fat (which is also an anti-inflammatory, that helped her digestive issues). As well, she was taking a multi-vitamin that had a metabolic boosting effect (see product resource guide).

When Kristine first started, her body mass index (BMI) was 30.3, which is considered obese. Her high BMI rating dramatically increased her risk of heart disease and type 2 diabetes. I am happy to report that Kristine's BMI is now considered normal at 24.8. She is fit, energetic and a vibrant looking woman.

7

Protein 101

"Take care of your body. It's the only place you have to live."

Jim Rohn,
American businessman, author, speaker and philosopher

Protein is the second macronutrient that you require in your daily diet. Protein is derived from building blocks called amino acids. Each protein is formed from the bonding of various amino acids into configurations. There are 20 amino acids in total. Out of the 20 amino acids, 11 are non-essential, which means your body can make them. The remaining nine must be derived from the food you consume on a daily basis (see table on page 149). Similar to the alphabet that can form a variety of long and short words, the different configurations of the amino acid structures are the building units for literally hundreds of protein varieties in the body.

A core constituent of the diet, protein serves as one of the major foundations for health, repair and replenishment. Our muscles, skin, hair and connective tissue are all made up of protein. Protein is also involved in many of the body's important chemical messengers such as enzymes, neurotransmitters and hormones.

Proteins are often deemed as "complete" or "incomplete," depending on their amino acid make-up. For example, animal proteins (meat, fish, poultry, milk, cheese and eggs) contain all nine essential amino acids and are considered complete, high-quality, absorbable options. Examples of incomplete proteins are legumes, nuts, seeds and grains. As you will soon discover, vegetarians can achieve proper protein intake by knowing the basics of where and how to get all of their amino acids. Similar to carbohydrates, proteins contain four calories per gram.

The Two Camps of Protein

When it comes to protein and weight loss, I normally see two camps of people. There is the first camp which consists of people who do not eat enough protein and are over-doing it on the wrong type of carbohydrates. These individuals are the "grab a muffin or toast for breakfast and eat rice, pasta or potatoes for dinner" kind of people. As you now know from the previous chapter, over-consuming the wrong type of carbohydrate will over-ring the insulin bell, and unless you are a star athlete constantly burning up fuel, you will gain weight.

The second camp of weight-loss seekers are those who have been lured by the recent high-protein diet draws and are eating too much protein in an attempt to take off the weight. Red meat, chicken, fish, turkey and other protein sources become the main source of fuel they rely on. Certain diets on the market go to a dangerous extreme with their carbohydrate restriction of 20 to 30 grams per day with no fruits allowed! While this technique results in temporary weight loss, similar to an extreme caloric restriction, an extreme restriction of carbohydrates will result in a backlash effect making future weight-loss attempts even more difficult. Remember, the body needs protein for weight loss, to build muscle, etc., but it does *not* want it as its primary source of fuel. It leaves that role up to our first macronutrient low-glycemic index (GI) carbohydrates.

Essential and Non-Essential Amino Acids

Essential	Non-Essential
Histadine	Alanine
Isoleucine	Arginine
Leucine	Asparagine
Valine	Aspartic Acid
Methionine	Cysteine
Phenylalanine	Glutamic Acid
Threonine	Glutamine
Tryptophan	Glycine
Lysine	Proline
	Serine
	Tyrosine

Glucagon: Insulin's Opposite

I can easily understand why people become so confused about how to lose weight and feel overwhelmed. I can also understand how gratifying it can be to go for an extremely high-protein diet and lose weight fast. Losing six to eight pounds per week can be a very attractive offer! Yet, I must reiterate a true and familiar motto: slow and steady always (and I mean *always*!) wins the race. If you are in hormonal balance from eating the proper amount of all three macronutrients (carbohydrates, proteins and fat), you will lose a considerable amount of weight per week and will keep it off for good. The major objective of *The Last 15* is permanent, not temporary results. My goal is for this to be your absolute last weight-loss attempt. Furthermore, if you feel the pounds creeping up again, or you fall off the health wagon when on vacation or during a stressful time, you now have the nutritional tools to take off any extra pounds and maintain your goal weight. The dance we have with food is constant: we overdo it on occasion and then balance it out (eat slightly less, work out, drink water, etc.). Figuring out how to master the dance is the key to enjoying your food, your health and your life.

For proteins this question begs to be answered: why do people lose weight when they go on high-protein diets? What is happening in the body that causes this to occur? In short, the answer to this very good question is glucagon. Glucagon is a pancreatic hormone that has the opposite effect to insulin. It is the delicate interplay between insulin and glucagon that determines whether your body stores or burns calories.

As we learned in the previous chapter, insulin is a store-and-save hormone that removes sugar (glucose) from the system and stores it as glycogen and fat. This process makes it much more difficult for the body to mobilize the body's fat stores. As insulin's opposite, glucagon is a mobilizing hormone and converts stored carbohydrates (glycogen) into glucose to be used for energy. In addition, glucagon also triggers the release of fat from the fat cells to be used as energy. Therefore, when insulin and glucagon are working in balance, weight-loss occurs, cravings subside, energy is increased and you enter a disease-prevention mode. In addition to causing excess weight gain, an over-secretion of insulin also contributes to inflammation, heart disease, high cholesterol and type 2 diabetes.

Let's face it: we love our carbohydrates! They are always available. Proteins are not as easy to obtain as carbohydrates and often take a little more thinking and planning ahead. That is why one of your *Last 15* mantras at every meal should be, "What is my protein source?" Keep in mind, carbohydrates have a storage depot in the body called glycogen. Glycogen can be stored in the liver and muscles and then called upon hours and even days later to be used as fuel. In contrast, proteins cannot be stored in the body. This is one of the fundamental reasons why you need to be able to identify your protein source at every meal: proteins constantly need to be replenished.

You do not need to concern yourself with weighing proteins or counting grams; I will be outlining simple ways to eyeball your food to estimate the amounts you are eating. However, you do need to be able to identify your protein source at all meals. Keep in mind, *The Last 15* is *not* a high-protein diet. High-protein diets can be dangerous to your health in the long run. High protein diets trigger the production of acidic substances called ketones. In an attempt to rid itself of the ketones, the body increases its urinary output. Although this may initially show up as pounds lost, it is water, not fat, that you're losing. If high-protein diets are followed long term, the body begins to break down muscle in a state called ketosis to urgently provide blood sugar for the brain. Ketosis is a state where the body is burning its own fat for fuel. In addition to feeling lethargic, there are other long-term consequences that can arise from over-consuming proteins and burning fat as fuel.

- **Kidney failure** Consuming too much protein puts a significant strain on the kidneys.
- **High cholesterol** High-protein diets consisting of red meat, whole dairy products and other high-fat foods have been linked to high cholesterol.
- **Osteoporosis and kidney stones** High-protein diets cause individuals to lose more calcium. Calcium acts as a buffer to the system that is overly acidic from eating too many high-protein foods.
- **Cancer** High-protein diets can increase the risks of cancer due to the restriction of high anti-oxidant rich foods such as colorful fruits and vegetables and whole grains.

In order to prevent a state of ketosis from kicking in, the body requires a minimum of 80 to 100 grams of carbohydrates per day.

How Much Protein Is Enough?

There is no greater debate in the athletic world than how much protein you require on a daily basis. There are a number of recommendations and calculations. On closer inspection, the daily intake of protein depends on your age and activity level. For example, weight trainers and teenagers require more protein than sedentary individuals.

When first starting to lose weight, I am an advocate of temporarily consuming more protein (30 percent of total calories consumed) in order to drag down insulin levels. This is what the first 30 days to re-setting your metabolic code is designed to do. The general principle is to halt the promotion of excess insulin secretion (which stores fat) and boost the amount of glucagon secretion (which breaks down fat). Once you start losing and/or reach your goal weight, you can slowly decrease your protein intake, all the while keeping your energy up and weight down. Even so, it is important to have a protein source at every meal to avoid the hypoglycemic effect (low blood sugar), to cut cravings, and to feel full and satisfied.

There are a few calculations that you can use to deterimine your protein intake. I recommend going by total percentage of calories per day. In other words, it is safe and within normal limits to consume 20 to 30 percent of your total calories per day from optimal protein sources such as lean meats, fish, chicken, egg whites and dairy products. During the 30 days to re-setting your metabolic code, in order to jump-start weight loss, the amount of protein you consume daily should be 30 pecent of your total daily calories. Following the first 30 (which you may be on for longer if you have more weight to lose), you can bring your protein intake down to 20 to 25 percent of your total daily calories. Keep in mind that some indiviudals who are extremely insulin sensitive, e.g., type 2 diabetics and chronic dieters, do better on a slightly higher protein intake in the long term.

So, in a nutshell, if you are a female consuming 1500 calories per day on the 30 days to re-setting your metabolic code, your total protein intake would be 30 percent of the total calories consumed.

1500 x 0.30 = 450 calories

Since 1 gram of protein = 4 calories, divide protein calories by 4. Your daily protein intake should be approximately 112.5 grams of protein.

If you are a female consuming 1500 calories per day and you are not on the 30 days to re-setting your metabolic code, your daily protien intake should be anywhere from 20 to 25 percent. Your calculations would look like this:

1500 x 0.20 = 300 calories from protein

= 300 calories / 4

= 75 grams of protein

You can easily consume this amount of protein each day. For example, a scoop of protein powder (20 to 25 grams of protein) in your morning shake, tuna on a salad at lunch (6 ounces of tuna = 40 grams of protein), a yogurt for a snack (approximately 6 grams) and a chicken breast with stir-fried vegetables for dinner (1 chicken breast = 30 grams of protein).

Protein Options

It is important to keep in mind that foods are classified according to the major macronutrient they contain. For example, a 3.5-ounce chicken breast does contain some fat, but it is mostly protein and is classified as a protein. The list below will highlight the foods that contain significant amounts of protein (beef, chicken, fish, turkey, eggs, soy and dairy), and other foods that contain less such as nuts and seeds.

On average, active women require four to six ounces of protein per meal, while active men require five to seven ounces of protein per meal. Snacks should contain approximately five to 10 grams of protein. (Please note: one ounce = 28 grams.)

Beef

- Hamburger patty, 4 ounces = 28 grams protein
- Steak, 6 ounces = 42 grams protein
- Most other cuts of beef, 1 ounce = 7 grams protein

Chicken

- Chicken breast, 3.5 ounces = 30 grams protein
- Chicken thigh, average size = 10 grams protein
- Drumstick = 11 grams protein
- Wing = 6 grams protein
- Chicken meat, 4 ounces = 35 grams protein

Fish

- Most fish filets or steaks = 22 grams protein
- Tuna, 6-ounce can = 40 grams protein

Pork

- Pork chop, average = 22 grams protein
- Pork loin or tenderloin, 4 ounces = 29 grams protein
- Ham, 3-ounce serving = 19 grams protein
- Bacon, 1 slice = 3 grams protein
- Canadian-style bacon (back bacon), 1 slice = 5–6 grams protein

Eggs and Dairy

- Egg, large = 6 grams protein
- Milk, 1 cup = 8 grams protein
- Cottage cheese, ½ cup = 15 grams protein
- Yogurt, 1 cup = 8–12 grams protein, usually (check label)
- Soft cheeses (Mozzarella, Brie, Camembert), 1 ounce = 6 grams protein
- Medium cheeses (Cheddar, Swiss), 1 ounce = 7 or 8 grams protein
- Hard cheeses (Parmesan), 1 ounce = 10 grams protein

Beans (including soy)

- Tofu, ½ cup = 20 grams protein
- Tofu, 1 ounce = 2.3 grams protein
- Soymilk, 1 cup = 6–10 grams protein
- Most beans (black, pinto, lentils, etc.), ½ cup cooked = approximately 7–10 grams protein
- Soy beans, ½ cup cooked = 14 grams protein
- Split peas, ½ cup cooked = 8 grams protein

Nuts and Seeds

- Peanut butter, 2 tbsp. = 8 grams protein
- Almonds, ¼ cup = 8 grams protein
- Peanuts, ¼ cup = 9 grams protein
- Cashews, ¼ cup = 5 grams protein
- Pecans, ¼ cup = 2.5 grams protein
- Sunflower seeds, ¼ cup = 6 grams protein
- Pumpkin seeds, ¼ cup = 19 grams protein
- Flaxseeds,¼ cup = 8 grams protein

Frequently Asked Questions and Answers about Protein

Now that you are aware of the protein basics and how glucagon works, let's clear up any protein confusion you may still have.

Question: What type of protein powder should I take?

Answer: I am a major advocate of always having a high-quality protein powder on hand. I recommend a protein shake mixed with berries, milk (low-fat, soy or rice) or orange juice, and flaxseed oil for a quick-and-easy breakfast to start off your morning.

There are several types of protein powders that are widely available in health food stores including whey, soy, hemp, egg and rice protein. Protein powders can contain one of these, or a mixture of two types, such as soy and whey or whey and egg.

I prefer protein powders that are composed of whey isolate. Whey is derived from milk and is the most commonly used protein supplement. It contains nonessential and essential amino acids, as well as branch chain amino acids (BCAA). Whey is easily absorbed by your muscles and is extremely safe to use. There are two categories of whey protein powders: 1) concentrate protein and 2) isolate protein. The concentrate protein contains approximately 30 to 85 percent protein, whereas the whey isolate protein is a higher quality protein containing more than 90 percent protein. Whey isolate is also more easily absorbed by the body and contains less fat and lactose.

Benefits of whey protein include:

- Helps boost immunity
- Optimal source of amino acids
- Enhances muscle recovery after workouts and helps prevent muscle breakdown

Please refer to the product resource guide for my favorite chocolate and vanilla protein powder recommendations!

Question: What is kefir?

***Answer*:** Kefir is similar to yogurt in taste and texture and is created by adding cow's or goat's milk to kefir grains which then undergo the fermentation process. Kefir supplies a complete protein source and is also filled with minerals, enzyme and friendly micro-organisms. In fact, one cup of kefir contains 14 grams of protein. Its rich supply of friendly bacteria optimizes digestion and makes it beneficial in restoring the internal micro flora of the intestinal systems, which is especially helpful following anti-biotic therapy. This dairy product can be used as is or in all recipes wherever yogurt or sour cream are used, e.g., protein shakes, salad dressings and dips.

Question: What if I am a vegetarian?

***Answer*:** To quote Nobel Prize recipient and famous physicist Albert Einstein (1879-1955) "Nothing will benefit human health and increase chances for survival of life on Earth as much as the evolution to a vegetarian diet." Vegetarian diets have often been credited with lowering the risk of colon cancer, heart attack, high blood cholesterol, high blood pressure, prostate cancer and stroke. If you are a semi or complete vegetarian, rest assured, you can still meet all your protein needs during the 30 days to re-setting your metabolic code and after.

If you eat dairy, eggs or some form of fish, meeting your protein needs is extremely easy. If, however, you are a vegan who avoids all animal products, including meats, dairy products and eggs, you will need to combine a variety of incomplete proteins to form complete proteins (see table below).

Food Combinations to Create Complete Proteins

Combine Grains and Legumes	Combine Grains and Nuts/Seeds	Combine Legumes and Nuts/Seeds
Peanut butter on whole-wheat bread	Whole-wheat bun with sesame seeds	Humus (chickpeas and sesame paste)
Rice and beans	Breadsticks rolled with sesame seeds	Trail mix (peanuts and sunflower seeds)
Bean soup and a roll	Rice cakes with peanut butter	
Salad with chickpeas and cornbread		
Tofu-vegetable stir-fry over rice or pasta		
Vegetarian chili with bread		

Question: What about red meat?

***Answer*:** There are a few issues of concern when it comes to eating large quantities of red meat. For starters, red meat is high in saturated fat which can contribute to the clogging of arteries. An excess of red meat can also promote inflammation in the body (as does an over-consumption of alcohol, white sugar and processed foods). To top it off, red meat is very hard to break down and digest, and can be incredibly taxing on the digestive system.

In terms of disease risk, studies have shown red meat to increase the risk of a variety of cancers such as colorectal, breast and prostate cancer. In addition, red meat has been linked to an increase of inflammatory conditions, e.g., arthritis, heart disease, high cholesterol, and stroke.

If you enjoy red meat, for health reasons, it is best to eat it sparingly (one serving per week) and select cuts of meat that are leaner and lower in saturated fat. That said, if you are suffering from a specific condition or are at high risk of disease, it is best to eliminate red meat from the diet all together. Chicken, turkey, fish and soy, e.g. veggie burgers, are all terrific substitutes that can help satisfy any former meat lover.

Here are some additional recommendations to help keep your red meat selections as healthy as possible:

- Select lean meat and alternatives prepared with little or no added fat or salt.
- Trim the visible fat from meats.
- Use cooking methods such as roasting, baking or poaching that require little or no added fat.
- If you eat luncheon meats, sausages or prepackaged meats, choose those lower in salt (sodium) and fat. Also, try only to eat pre-packaged meats that are nitrite-free. Nitrites are chemical preservatives that give meat its pinkish hue, e.g. bologna, hot dogs. Unfortunately, nitrates, have also been shown to have carcinogenic (cancer-causing) effects. Stick to nitrate free options or imitation vegetarian options such as veggie hot dogs.

Question: What about tuna?

Answer: One of the most common questions that people ask when I am lecturing is, "Is tuna safe to eat?" Tuna is certainly among the most popular fish for families to enjoy. In fact, it appears in over 90 percent of households and makes up approximately 20 percent of all U.S. fish consumption. Children and pregnant women eat more than twice as much tuna as any other fish.

In recent years, there has been great controversy surrounding the consumption of tuna due to high mercury levels contained in the fish. In fact, the most common source of human exposure to mercury is due to the consumption of certain types of tuna. It is estimated that mercury levels in the environment have increased three to five times in the past century due to industrial operations such as pulp and paper processing, burning garbage and fossil fuels, mining operations and releases from dental offices. This mercury can spill into our waters and pollute our marine life.

The problem is that research and guidelines on how to safely eat tuna are not consistent and are ever-changing. If you love tuna but are concerned about the mercury content, I recommend eating canned light tuna packed in water rather than white albacore tuna, which is higher in mercury content. Light tuna is a mixture of tuna species and contains far less mercury. If albacore tuna is your favorite and you want to know how much is okay, the most recent guidelines suggest 6 ounces per week is the maximum you should consume. For pregnant or breastfeeding women and young children, my recommendation is to stick with light tuna. Please refer to the product resource section for a low mercury tuna option.

Question: Is farmed salmon safe to eat?

***Answer*:** In an attempt to avoid the mercury found in tuna, many fish lovers have turned to salmon as a healthy option. The upside of doing so is that salmon is full of protein and omega-3 heart-healthy fats. The downside is that farmed salmon is not as healthy as we once thought. According to several recent studies, farmed salmon contains unsafe levels of dioxins and PCBs. Dioxins and PCBs are chemicals formed by unwanted by-products in a variety of industrial processes. They are found throughout the environment, and fish accumulate them mostly from eating other fish and from fish feed. PCBs have not been used since the 1970s, but are still lingering because they persist in the environment for several years. Dioxins and PCBs have been linked to several serious health conditions such as liver damage, immune system suppression and developmental delay in children.

In a large scale study reported in 2004, the average dioxin level in farm-raised salmon was 11 times higher than in wild salmon. The study also reported the average PCB levels were 36.6 parts per billion (ppb) in farm-raised salmon, versus 4.75 ppb in wild salmon. In response to this study, the World Health Organization (WHO) released the following statement:

"WHO consider fish to be an important component of a nutritious diet, and that the risk of consuming contaminated fish must be weighed in view of the beneficial nutritive effects of fish. FAO and WHO plan to develop general guidance for such risk-benefit considerations, with the contamination of fish as case studies."

It is best to purchase "cleaner" salmon in the form of wild Atlantic salmon. I realize this option is more of a splurge, but with consumer demand and pressure, the price will soon fall. In addition to having a significantly lower toxic load, once you eat wild Atlantic salmon in the form of fillet or smoked salmon (lox), you will instantly notice the difference in color, taste and texture. The good news is, most canned salmon available in grocery stores is derived from wild sources.

Protein in a Nutshell

Before we move on to the following chapter on fats, it is important to re-cap the importance of protein. In order to keep insulin levels in check, a proper protein intake will facilitate the secretion of the hormone glucagon (insulin's opposite). Eating protein will fill you up, sustain energy levels, rebuild and repair muscle and is a must for metabolic boosting and weight loss.

Keep in mind that striking a balance with protein and carbohydrates is critical to your overall weight-loss success. You do not want to go too high with your protein intake (the body wants carbohydrates as the main source of fuel!), yet you do need enough protein to facilitate hormonal balance and weight loss.

Marg

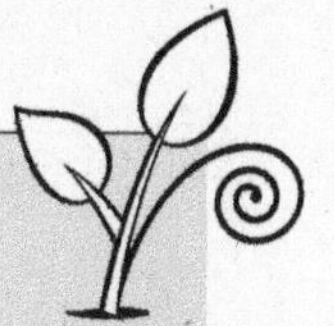

Age: 43

Starting weight: 172 pounds

Current weight: 148 pounds!

Marg is a busy lady. She owns seven food franchises, has 85 employees, two daughters, one husband and no time! With her busy schedule, the weight simply started to creep up on her. At age 43, she weighed in at 172 pounds and described her life as a "1 kilogram bag of M&M's, beer, drive-throughs and pre-packaged meals." Marg is a "pleaser," and hence tended always to do for others and did not take the time she needed for herself. With her faulty food choices and lack of exercise, Marg's health began to pay the price, both physically and mentally.

After trying numerous popular diets, Marg had simply had enough. She did not want to follow another temporary fad and was more interested in a way of eating that she could maintain for life. After a "light-bulb" moment about her health and wellness, Marg decided to finally say good-bye to the potato chips, fried foods, ice cream and white bread she was eating on a daily basis and opened the door to delicious and healthy eating. She now enjoys a variety of Last 15 foods such as low-fat cheese, berries, whole grains, and high-quality protein options such as chicken, fish and tasty omelets. In addition, during highly emotional times or times of stress, Marg also has a very supportive weight-loss "buddy," whom she leans on for extra motivation and encouragement. Marg has learned the importance of eating breakfast, listening to her body and making the time for health. I am thrilled to report that as I write this passage, Marg has lost over 23 pounds.

8

Fats 101

"Money is the most envied, but the least enjoyed. Health is the most enjoyed, but the least envied."

Charles Caleb Colton (1780-1832),
Writer for *British Sportsman*

Imagine this common scenario. You start off your day with a breakfast that consists of non-fat cereal and non-fat milk with banana slices, orange juice and a coffee with milk and sugar. Do you lose weight? Absolutely not! In fact, you gain weight, feel starving and shaky by 10 a.m. and continue your day feeling fatigued and eating sugar in the form of a variety of high-glycemic index (GI) carbohydrates! Not the best recipe for long-term weight loss results, is it?

Poor fat...this essential macronutrient is so misunderstood. From low-fat diets to an abundant amount of "fat free" foods—most people are dodging this precious macronutrient in an attempt to lose weight and keep it off for good. Do you need fat in the diet for weight loss, anti-inflammatory purposes, optimal health and functioning of every cell in the body? Absolutely! However, the key is to understand the difference between the good types of fat and the bad.

Prior to detailing which fats are "good" and which fats are "bad," it is important to point out that fats contain 9 calories for every 1 gram. This is more than double the calories in protein and carbohydrates, which have 4 calories in every 1 gram. Therefore, when it comes to fat, think of a "sprinkling." You do not need as much fat as you do carbohydrates and protein, but you certainly do need to eat a specific amount of the good fats daily.

Eating Licorice for Weight Loss?

About a year ago, I had a very excited client bring in a package of a popular red licorice. "Look at this", she exclaimed. "This licorice contains no fat! Yippee!" This means we can eat licorice on a diet, lose weight and feel great, right? Not so fast. The answer to this is two thumbs down.

If we think back to a few years ago, we can all remember the surge of low-fat diets. In grocery stores across the nation, products were slapped with "low fat" labels in an attempt to promote their weight-loss effects. Historically, this is how diets work. The latest fad diets such as a low-fat, high-protein or the grapefruit diet, for example, come in and out of favor, drawing in new weight-loss seekers. Although some of the diets offer sound nutritional advice, most have a "magic bullet" lure that has little to do with holistic nutrition. The result is that people usually lose weight temporarily, but as their motivation wanes and taste buds wander to more stimulating and exciting food, they drop their diet and gain back all of the weight they lost and then some. Does this sound familiar to you? Even today, the label of "low fat" appears to be a significant draw for consumers. In fact, a national survey conducted in 2000 by Booth Research Services for the Calorie Control Council revealed 188 million adult Americans (88 percent of the adult U.S. population) consume low- or reduced-fat foods and beverages. Don't be fooled by this! Keep in mind the ever-important Last 15 rule: if any diet drastically reduces or eliminates one of the three core macronutrients, it is *not* a sustainable diet. Knowing the facts and selecting healthy fat options is the key to health and permanent weight loss.

Let's call a spade a spade: fat tastes delicious! In fact, fat provides food products with a specific texture that satiates and makes food taste great. Without it, food is bland and needs something extra to improve flavor. So… if you are a food manufacturer and remove fat from a product in order to be able to market it as "low fat," what do you typically add to improve taste and appeal to consumers' taste buds? Sugar, of course! As you now know, eating too many high-GI products loaded with sugar and refined flours creates excess insulin, excess fat, intensifies cravings and causes energy to dip. Alas, eating licorice or any other food product whose first ingredient is sugar, high-fructose corn syrup or glucose is not the way to lose weight and feel great. In addition to avoiding misleading low-fat foods that are heavy on the sugar, eating high-quality fat options that satiate, are anti-inflammatory and are equally delicious is the proper path to losing weight.

Low-fat Diets and the Risk of Heart Disease and Cancer

Until recently, government agencies typically recommended low-fat diets as a preventative approach to heart disease and a variety of cancers. In fact, research shows that this simply is not the case. According to the largest study ever conducted designed to investigate if a low-fat diet reduces disease risk, the answer was a resounding no!

This $415 million dollar study followed 49,000 women aged 50 to 79 years of age for eight years. At the end of the study, those assigned to a low-fat diet had the same rates of breast cancer, colon cancer, heart attacks and strokes as compared to those not on a low-fat diet. Another study that investigated popular fad diets found that low-fat diets were the most ineffective for weight loss. Findings revealed that people who were on the low-fat diet actually lost the least amount of weight! Finally, in a study that appeared in the May, 2003 *New England Journal of Medicine*, researchers found that obese patients who were placed on a low-carbohydrate diet for six months lost more weight and scored better on cardiovascular and diabetes markers than those on a low-fat, calorie-restricted diet.

Participants in the low-carbohydrate group were not given a limit on total fat intake but were educated on the healthy types of fats, such as omega-3s. The low-fat group was limited to no more than 30 percent of caloric intake from fat. The results showed:

- The low-carbohydrate, higher-fat dieters lost an average of 13 pounds compared to 4 pounds for the low-fat group.
- Triglyceride levels (fats in the blood that can cause heart disease) were lowered by an average of 20 percent in the low-carbohydrate group vs. 4 percent in the low-fat group.
- Insulin sensitivity in non-diabetic people improved in those on the low-carbohydrate diet as opposed to the low-fat diet (fasting blood sugars reduced by 9 percent vs. 2 percent in the low-fat group).

The above study does not suggest that you should eliminate carbohydrates from the diet. As we saw in Chapter 6, "Carbohydrates 101," you definitely require low-GI carbohydrates in the form of vegetables, fruits and whole grains; they provide the fuel that runs your body. However, you must eat fat to lose fat, but it must be the right type of fat.

The Different Types of Fat

When lecturing, I always say, "Do not feel bad if you are confused about how to eat fats. There are several types of fats, and determining the good from the bad takes a little bit of information." Fats can be broken down into the following categories:

- Trans fatty acids
- Saturated fats
- Polyunsaturated fats
- Monounsaturated fats
- Essential fats

Trans Fatty Acids

Trans fatty acids are a specific type of fat formed when liquid vegetable oils are made into solid fats like shortening and hard margarine. Most of the trans fat in the typical North American diet are derived from commercially baked and fried foods that are made with vegetable shortening, some margarine (especially hard margarines) or oils containing partially hydrogenated oils and fats. French fries, donuts, pastries, muffins, croissants, cookies, crackers, chips and other snack foods are typically high in trans fatty acids. In fact, nearly all fried or commercially baked goods have some trans fats. The trans fat content of these foods may be as high as 45 to 50 percent of the fat.

As a general rule, essential fats such as flaxseed oil are fairly fragile and have a shorter shelf life than trans fats. For example, once opened, flaxseed oil will only last in the refrigerator for approximately three months; after that it needs to be discarded as it can become rancid. While essential fats are terrific for overall health and wellness, they are not the best option if you are in the food business.

Let's say you are a food manufacturer and you want fat in your food product to achieve the proper taste and texture. Of course, time and ingredients are costly and you do not want to be clearing items off the shelf and throwing them out after three months. What is the solution to this potentially costly problem? Flood that little fat molecule with hydrogen, chemically change the shape of it and—voila—you have a product with a shelf-life of five to seven years! Food technologists alter the chemical structure of polyunsaturated liquid fat (vegetable oil) from a round to a straight chain shape. This process is called hydrogenation and involves flooding a polyunsaturated fat with an abundant amount of hydrogen at a high temperature. In other words, hydrogenation straightens out the molecules so they can lie closer together and become solid rather than liquid. This is terrific news for food manufacturers, but terrible news for cholesterol levels and a host of other health issues.

As you probably know, eating trans fatty acids can have tremendously negative effects on your health. These fake fats raise total blood cholesterol levels and LDL ("bad") cholesterol and lower HDL ("good") cholesterol levels. This in turn can increase your risk of coronary heart disease, which leads to heart attack and increases the risk of stroke.

As of January 1, 2006, packaged food products must list the trans fats content on the Nutrition Facts panel. The amount of trans fats per serving of food will appear under the "Total Fat" section of the label. The Food and Drug Administration (FDA) requires that the amount of trans fat in a serving be listed on a separate line under saturated fat on the "Nutrition Facts" panel (see sample label on page 206). However, trans fat does not have to be listed if the total fat in a food is less than 0.5 gram (or ½ gram) per serving and no claims are made about fat, fatty acids or cholesterol content. If it is not listed, a footnote is required stating that the food is "not a significant source of trans fat." In addition, food manufacturers are allowed to list amounts of trans fat with less than 0.5 gram (½ g) as 0 (zero) on the Nutrition Facts panel. As a result, consumers may see a few products that list 0 gram trans fat on the label, while the ingredient list will have "shortening" or "partially hydrogenated vegetable oil" on it. This means the food contains very small amounts (less than 0.5 g) of trans fat per serving. However, it's important to know that if you eat four servings or more of the specific food product per day, you will be consuming too much trans fat.

For those food products that do not yet list the amount of trans fatty acids on the labels, you can determine the amount on your own. Simply add up the values for saturated, polyunsaturated and monounsaturated fats. If the number is less than the "Total fats" shown on the label, the unaccounted fat is derived from trans fat.

In addition to trans fats now being listed on labels, as of April 2004, the FDA food advisory committee voted in favor of recommending that daily trans fatty acid intake be reduced to less than 1 percent of energy (e.g., 2 grams per 2000 kcal diet/day).

Trans fatty acids (TFAs) are also found in many fried foods in fast food chains such as chicken nuggets and French fries. If for example you continue to have that doughnut for lunch (3.2 g TFA) and large fries at dinner (6.8 g TFA), you may be eating as much as 10 grams of trans fatty acids per day! Since it is difficult, if not impossible, to determine the oil the fast food chain has been using for frying, you should simply avoid fast food and deep fried food items.

Keep in mind that not all trans fatty acids are bad. In fact, there are naturally occurring trans fatty acids found in beef, lamb and dairy products that may be beneficial to health (research is still warranted). It is the trans fatty acids found in packaged and processed foods, deep fried foods and fast food that is harmful and therefore needs to be eliminated.

"On Dec. 5, 2006, New York City's board of health approved a ban on trans fats in all restaurants across the city."

Saturated Fat

Saturated fats are usually solid, or almost solid, at room temperature. These types of fat are found in animal products such as butter, cheese, whole milk, ice cream, cream and fatty meats. In fact, the Center for Science in the Public Interest describes cheese as America's number one source of saturated fat, adding that the average American ate 30 pounds

(13.6 kg) of cheese in the year 2000, up from 11 pounds (5 kg) in 1970. Saturated fats can also be found in some vegetable oils such as coconut, palm, and palm kernel oils.

While saturated fats are not considered as bad as trans fatty acids, excessive consumption of saturated fats can raise the level of the bad cholesterol known as low-density lipoprotein (LDL). High LDL levels (above 160mg/dl) increase the risk of heart disease because they keep cholesterol in blood circulation and carry it to the arteries to be deposited. In addition to raising LDL levels, research has also demonstrated that eating too many of the wrong fats such as saturated and trans fatty acids increases inflammation in the body. According to a study appearing in *The American Journal of Clinical Nutrition*, within an hour of eating a fatty meal, participants experienced increases in inflammatory proteins associated with heart disease. Levels remained elevated for as long as three to four hours after the meal. Chronic inflammatory reactions have been linked to numerous ill health issues such as heart disease, dementia and Alzheimer's. Any time you have an "itis" in the body (colitis, bursitis, etc.), the root cause is inflammatory. Pay attention to the percentage of saturated fat on the Nutrition Fact Panel and avoid or limit any foods that are high (over 20 percent) in saturated fat.

One of the questions I commonly am asked about saturated fats is why the French, one of the largest cheese consumers in the world, also have one of the lowest rates of heart disease, obesity and high cholesterol. The answer to the "French Paradox" is very simple—portion size. In fact, a group of scientists from France's CNRS scientific research institute and the University of Pennsylvania decided to investigate the winning weight-loss ways of the French. Researchers weighed portions at 11 similar restaurants in Paris and Philadelphia and found the following:

- The average portion size in Paris was 25 percent smaller than in Philadelphia.
- Chinese restaurants in Philadelphia served dishes that were 72 percent larger than in Parisian Chinese food restaurants.

A comparison between local supermarkets found:

- A candy bar in Philadelphia was 41 percent larger than the same candy bar in Paris.
- A soft drink was 53 percent larger and a hot dog was 63 percent larger.

When North Americans indulge, they tend to overdo it on portion size. The French nibble and indulge without over-consuming. It is almost as if they have been trained from childhood on how far they can cheat with food without paying the price in excess pounds. In my last book, *The Natural Makeover Diet,* I strongly encourage readers to slow down while eating and to eat until they are sufficiently satisfied not stuffed. Why? It takes 20 minutes for the stretch receptors in your stomach to say to your brain, "Hey, I'm full. That is enough food, thank you!" Taking smaller bites, chewing your food, using your utensils and slowing down will all cause you to feel fuller and to eat less.

In addition to smaller portion sizes, the French get more exercise. As most Parisians will tell you, they love to walk! Rarely do they use transportation as we do. Instead, they simply step outside their front door and walk and—presto—they start to instantly boost their metabolism and overall health.

Polyunsaturated Fats

Polyunsaturated fat is found in vegetable oils such as safflower, corn, sunflower and soybean. This type of fat remains liquid at room temperature. Although people used to think of vegetable oils as healthy fats, this is not the case. While polyunsaturated fats indeed do lower the level of bad cholesterol (LDL), they are also believed to lower good cholesterol, known as high-density lipoprotein (HDL). HDL is known as the "good" cholesterol because it has the opposite effect of LDL (the "bad" cholesterol). HDL carries plaque away from the arterial wall to the liver and out of the body. As you will discover in the following section on essential fats, eating too many omega-6 polyunsaturated fats in the form of refined vegetable oils decreases the amount of a necessary fat called omega-3 and can contribute to excess inflammation. In addition, these types of oils are very sensitive to heat and light, and they oxidize readily, which makes them susceptible to rancidity. While vegetable oils should be kept in dark bottles and stored in the fridge, they are mostly refined and found in clear bottles on grocery store shelves.

Monounsaturated Fats

Monounsaturated fats are among the healthiest fats in the world. In fact, the Mediterranean approach to food contains a significant amount of monounsaturated fats, all the while offering the benefits of a lower risk of heart disease. Monounsaturated fats can be found in olive oil (73 percent), rapeseed oil (60 percent), hazel nuts (50 percent), almonds (35 percent), Brazil nuts (26 percent), cashews (28 percent), avocados (12 percent), sesame seeds (20 percent) and pumpkin seeds (16 percent).

As you can see, olive oil contains the highest amount of monounsaturated fats of all the edible oils. Olive oil is ideal as a cooking oil as it has the highest oxidation threshold: that means it remains stable at higher temperatures and does not easily become hydrogenated or saturated. The best type of olive oil to buy is that labeled "extra-virgin," made from the first pressing of the olives. This oil is very flavorful and can be used for cooking or in salad dressings. All oils should be stored in dark, cool places.

The health benefits of monounsaturated fats are numerous and include:

- Lowering cholesterol and risk of heart disease
- May offer protection against certain types of cancers such as breast cancer and colon cancer
- Is high in vitamin E, a very potent anti-oxidant vitamin
- Cold press olive oil is filled with a variety of phytochemicals (plant nutrients which boost immune system function)
- Preliminary research shows substituting olive oil for saturated fat in

your diet can translate into a small but significant loss of both body weight and fat mass without changing anything else about your diet or increasing your physical activity

It is unclear if the health benefits of olive oil are linked to its high content of monounsaturated fat or the abundance of polyphenols (anti-oxidants) in the oil. Nonetheless, this superfood should certainly be included in your daily diet.

Essential Fats

You have likely heard a lot about omega-3 fatty acids in the news in recent years. When researchers and scientists identify a food source that offers significant health benefits, (usually through what is called a double-blind research study, the gold standard of research), the public begins to see these food items pop up on grocery store shelves, on labels, and in various advertisements. Green tea, white tea, omega-3, probiotics and flaxseeds are among the recently popularized foods. There is now an abundant amount of research that demonstrates the health benefits and the disease-preventing properties of omega-3 fats. And yes, these essential fats can even help with weight loss!

We call these *essential* fatty acids because they are vital for health and cannot be produced by the body. Every living cell in the body needs essential fatty acids to rebuild and produce new cells. In fact, the cell membrane, the barrier that surrounds the cell and allows the influx of nutrients and the export of toxins, is comprised of fatty acids. To perform these functions at an optimal level and maintain health, the cell membrane must maintain its integrity and fluidity. Cells without an intact cellular membrane lose the ability to properly communicate with each other and can create the platform on which ill health and disease flourish. Researchers believe the type of fat we consume in our diet has a significant effect on our cellular membranes. In other words, diets high in saturated fats and trans fatty acids produce cell membranes that are hard and less flexible, while diets high in essential healthy fats have more fluidity to their cellular membranes.

Essential fats are also classified as polyunsaturated fats, but can be differentiated from the refined vegetables oils that create an environment in which inflammation can occur. There are two basic categories of essential fatty acids.

1. Omega-3 fatty acids called alpha-linolenic acid (ALA)
2. Omega-6 fatty acids called linoleic acid

Once eaten, the body converts ALA to EPA (eicosapentaenoic acid) and DHA (docosahexaenoic acid), the two types of omega-3 fatty acids more readily used by the body.

Although a certain amount of omega-6 and omega-3 are necessary in the diet, a problem arises when too many omega-6 fats are consumed. The balance of omega-6 to omega-3 is very important and they work together much like a teeter-totter. In other words, if an individual has too much of one kind of essential fat, they will become deficient in the other. Consuming too much polyunsaturated fat in the form of processed vegetable oils creates an imbalance in the ratio of omega-6 essential fatty acids to omega-3 essential fatty acids. The typical American diet tends to contain 11 to 30 times more omega-6 fatty acids than omega-3 fatty acids. The ideal ratio is approximately one to one to two to one (omega-6! omega-3). Many researchers believe this imbalance is a significant factor in the rising rate of inflammatory disorders.

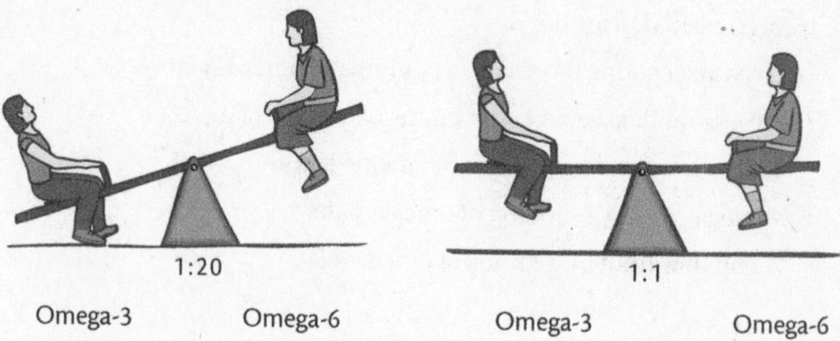

Research has identified many common conditions and disorders linked to the deficiency of omega-3 essential fatty acids. Examples include:

- Depression
- Attention deficit disorder
- Cardiovascular disease
- Type 2 diabetes
- Fatigue
- Dry, itchy skin
- Brittle hair and nails
- Inability to concentrate
- Joint pain
- Inflammatory conditions such as arthritis, colitis, etc.

It should be noted that essential fatty acids are highly concentrated in the brain and appear to be particularly important for cognitive and behavioral function. In fact, infants who do not get enough omega-3 fatty acids from their mothers during pregnancy are at risk for developing vision and nerve problems. Research has also clearly shown omega-3 fats to be beneficial in boosting metabolic function and burning fat. Please see the section on fish oils in Chapter 9 for more detail.

Optimal omega-3 food sources are flaxseed oil, omega-3 eggs, deepwater fish and fish oil, walnuts and walnut oil, almonds, sesame seeds soybeans and omega-3 fortified foods. Optimal sources of omega-6 are found in unrefined foods such as raw nuts, seeds, legumes, borage oil, grapeseed oil and primrose oil.

- Two tablespoons flaxseeds = 3.5 grams of omega-3 fats
- 1 teaspoon flaxseed oil = 2.5 grams of omega-3 fats
- 4 ounces salmon =1.5 grams of omega-3 fats
- 1 omega-3 egg = 3–400mg of omega-3 fats
- ¼ cup of walnuts = 2 grams of omega-3 fat

On September 8, 2006, the U.S. Food and Drug Administration gave "qualified health claim" status to eicosapentaenoic acid (EPA) and docosahexaenoic acid (DHA) omega-3 fatty acids, stating that "supportive but not conclusive research shows that consumption of EPA and DHA omega-3 fatty acids may reduce the risk of coronary heart disease.

Common Sources of Fat

Family Name	Common Name	Food Source
omega-9	Oleic acid	Canola, olive, and peanut oils, animal products, avocado
omega-6	Linoleic acid	Corn, safflower, soybean, cottonseed and sunflower oils (the pro-inflammatory oils) Borage, black current and primrose oils (the anti-inflammatory oils that contain GLA)
	Arachadonic acid	Animal products
omega-3	Alpha-linolenic acid	Canola and soybean oils, some nuts, flaxseed, green leafy vegetables, blueberries
	Eicosapentaenoic acid (EPA)	Fish
	Docosahexainoic acid (DHA)	Fish

Flaxseed Oil or Fish Oil?

I am commonly asked if it is better to supplement with fish oils or flaxseed oil. While flaxseed oil is a terrific oil to use in salad dressings or in a morning shake, its conversion to a more absorbable form of essential fat is not as efficient as fish oil. Research suggests you need to take almost 10 times the amount of flaxseed oil to get the equivalent amount of DHA and EPA found in fish oils. Typically, this means approximately 7.2 grams of flaxseed oil equals one gram of fish oil.

While there is no harm in taking flaxseed oil and fish oil to boost your omega-3 intake, if you are taking supplements, I recommend taking the fish oil supplement and using flaxseed oil in recipes and shakes. Flaxseeds offer wonderful options: you can use flaxseed oil in salad dressings or sprinkle ground flaxseeds into your morning shake, cereal, on a salad or in juice. But flaxseed alone is not enough. Although the major type of fat present in flaxseed oil, ALA, can be converted to EPA and DHA (the two types of omega-3 fat more readily absorbed by the body), for the majority of people, the conversion appears to be inefficient. For example, fish oil has been shown to have anti-inflammatory effects for conditions such as rheumatoid arthritis, while the effects of flaxseed oil on inflammation are inconclusive. Fish oil has also been shown to reduce platelet aggregation (the stickiness of your blood cells) which is a risk factor for heart disease, while flaxseed oil did not demonstrate the same results.

In short, flaxseed oil or ground flax seeds are a wonderful addition to any diet and should be used daily. There are some health benefits such as reducing cholesterol and aiding with constipation associated with ground flaxseeds and flaxseed oil. However, they should not be relied on as a source of omega-3 due to their inefficient conversion to EPA and DHA. When using flaxseed oil, keep in mind it should never be heated. This type of oil is not suitable for cooking and should always be stored in an opaque, airtight container in the refrigerator or freezer. If the oil has a noticeable odor, it is probably rancid and should be discarded.

Whole flaxseeds can be purchased at most bulk food or health food stores. The outer husk of flaxseeds is very hard and difficult to crack when chewing. Because of this, whole flaxseeds must be ground up in a coffee grinder, food processor or blender in order for the body to digest them when eaten. If not, whole flaxseeds will pass right through the body undigested and you will lose all of their nutritional advantage. By grinding them up, the body will benefit from the fiber, essential oils and lignans (beneficial plant chemicals) that are present. I recommend grinding your flaxseeds quite fine for the best palatability. To ensure freshness, after grinding, store your flaxseeds in an airtight, dark container. Ground flax stays fresh and safe to eat for 90 days. Keep in mind that there is no nutritional difference between brown flaxseed and golden or yellow flaxseed. Both types of flaxseeds offer the goodness of fiber, phytonutrients and omega-3 fats, but often it is easier to find brown flaxseeds than golden.

Flaxseed Oil Salad Dressing

Ingredients:

extra virgin olive oil	2 tbsp.
flaxseed oil	1 tbsp.
white balsamic vinegar	1 tbsp.
lemon juice	1 tsp.
capers	2 tbsp.
fresh chopped garlic	½ tsp.

Salt and freshly ground black pepper to taste

Directions:

In a small bowl, whisk together the olive oil, flaxseed oil, vinegar, lemon juice, chopped garlic and capers. Season with salt and pepper.

Note: If you are on a blood thinning medication or about to go for surgery, talk to your doctor prior to supplementing with fish oils.

"Low Fat" Labels

Consumers often see the words "low fat" on labels, but what does this claim really mean? According to the U.S. food labeling regulations implemented in 1994, there a number of claims that can indicate a reduction in fat content. They are outlined below.

"Low Fat" Claims on Labels

- *Fat-free*: less than 0.5g fat per serving
- *Low-fat*: 3g fat or less per serving size
- *Reduced or less fat*: 25% less fat than the food it is being compared to
- *Percent fat free*: A product bearing this claim must be a low-fat or a fat-free product. In addition, the claim must accurately reflect the amount of fat present in 100 g of the food. Thus, if a food contains 2.5 g fat per 50 g, the claim must be "95 percent fat free."
- *Low saturated fat*: 1g or less and 15% or less of calories from saturated fat
- *Trans fat free*: Less than 0.5g of trans fat per serving
- *Lite/Light*: 50% less fat or one third fewer calories than the regular product

"Low Fat" Claims for Meat, Poultry, Seafood and Game Meats

- *Lean*: less than 10g fat, 4.5g or less saturated fat and less than 95mg cholesterol per 100 grams of meat, poultry or seafood.
- *Extra lean*: less than 5g fat, less than 2g saturated fat and less than 95 mg cholesterol per serving and per 100g of meat, poultry or seafood.

Calories

- *Calorie-free*: less than 5 calories per serving or reference amount
- *Low-calorie*: 40 calories or less per reference serving size
- *Reduced or fewer calories*: 25% or less calories per serving than regular product

What about Dairy Products?

High-quality dairy products can quickly add calcium, protein and vitamin B to your diet; I recommend eating them for weight loss and weight maintenance. Unlike a processed food that is labeled "low fat" and is filled with sugar, low-fat dairy products are indeed lower in saturated fat and will not trigger an excess of insulin. In other words, this is the one time where I encourage people to opt for the low-fat option. Even so, it is always wise to be a conscientious label reader. There are certain low-fat dairy products, e.g. yogurts with added syrupy fruits, that are high in sugar. In order to know how much sugar is in your food, the rule of thumb is one teaspoon of sugar equals four grams. Therefore, if a yogurt contains 12 grams of sugar per serving, that is three teaspoons! In order to determine if a food item is loaded to the brim with added sugar, check the ingredients list. If the first or second word is *sugar, sucrose, high-fructose corn syrup, corn syrup, confectioner's sugar, corn sweeteners, dextrose, glucose, fructose, maltose, molasses, honey, brown sugar, fruit and juice concentrate, invert sugar, cane sugar, raw sugar, galactose, lactose, levulose and/or maple sugar*, beware of the sugar content!

When grocery shopping for dairy products, look for those that are low in sugar and are low in fat, e.g., low-fat, fat-free or reduced-fat alternatives. A low-fat dairy product has less than 3 grams of fat per serving. Choose skim milk over whole milk and low-fat or fat-free sour cream over whole sour cream. Read package labels carefully. Look for the grams of total fat and saturated fat per serving when you compare similar products.

Here are some easy ways to incorporate low-fat dairy products into your diet:

- Choose skim milk, reduced-fat cheeses and lower fat milk desserts, such as ice milk or frozen yogurt.
- Top your vegetables with fat-free or low-fat yogurt or shredded, fat-free cheese. Remember, full-fat cheese has big flavor and big fat content! An ounce or two (1 ounce equals your thumb or four dice) can be tasty and satisfying at the same time.
- Plain yogurt mixed with fresh fruit makes a quick and easy snack. Since plain yogurt has no added sugars, it's the best choice to reduce your

sugar and calorie intake. Plus, you get added fiber and antioxidants from fresh fruit such as strawberries, blueberries or banana slices.

- When buying dairy products, go organic.
- Avoid cream soups and heavy cream sauces.

If you do find you have a reaction to eating dairy products, you should try eating goat cheese. Not only does goat cheese offer a delicious taste that is fantastic in salads, it is much more easily digested than dairy products made from cow's milk.

Tips for Consuming Fats

- Eat a sprinkling of fats: 10 nuts, 1 to 2 teaspoons of olive oil, ¼ avocado, etc.
- Eliminate processed trans fatty acids from your diet. Read the Nutrition Facts panel on the label for the presence of trans fats.
- Minimize saturated fats such as full-fat cheeses or red meat.
- When selecting dairy products, go for low-fat (but watch for the sugar content in products such as yogurt).
- Eliminate omega-6 refined vegetable oils.
- Maximize monounsaturated fats such as extra virgin olive oil, almonds, cashews and avocados.
- Maximize omega-3 fats in the diet in the form of fortified foods (eggs, juice, bread), nuts (almonds, walnuts), sesame seeds, cold water fish, flaxseeds and flaxseed oil and fish oil.

As you have just discovered, healthy fats are critical to overall health and wellness and are part of an effective weight-loss and weight-maintenance diet. On average, healthy fats should make up approximately 25 to 30 percent of the total calories you consume each day. If you are a female who consumers 1500 calories per day, you would calculate your daily fat intake as follows:

1500 x 0.25 = 375 calories from fats.

Since 1 grams of fat = 9 calories, divide fat calories by 9. Your daily fat intake should be approximately 41 grams of fat.

You can easily attain this by having a tablespoon of flaxseed oil in a morning shake (14 grams of fat), 10 almonds for snack (7 grams of fat), 3 thin avocado slices on a pita sandwich at lunch (5 grams of fat) and using 1 tablespoon of olive oil to cook a stir-fry with (13 grams of fat).

Keep in mind that to maintain your weight-loss, your optimal daily caloric intake of macronutrients in the proper percentages are:

- 25–30% lean proteins
- 25–30% essential fats
- 40–50% low-GI carbohydrates

An exception may occur during the 30 days to re-setting your metabolic code, when your protein intake will be slightly higher to get insulin secretion in check.

Mary, Elisa, Elena and Victoria: The Fabulous Housewives

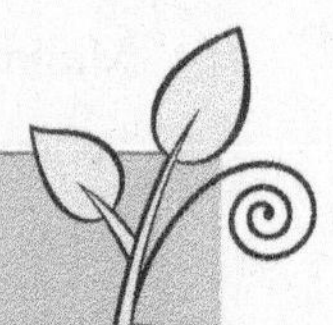

Recently, I met a woman at my son's school who was interested in losing weight and getting her high cholesterol levels under control. She mentioned that she had a few friends who also needed to lose weight and thought a group setting would work. Perfect! I thought, the more the merrier. I also knew that having each other as a support system would increase the weight-loss success they were about to experience.

When I first met these women their affable personalities and sense of humor were infectious. In short, they were a riot and I affectionately called the group "the fabulous housewives." After taking a detailed health history of all four women, I was stunned to find out that between them, they have 16 children! One of these lovely women has five children under the age of eight, while another is a single mom with four children (two teenagers and two toddlers) and is struggling to make ends meet. We decided to meet once a week after we had all tucked our kids into bed to review food journals, have a weekly weigh-in and to answer any questions in the evening.

I instantly knew that these women were fed up with the excess weight they gained during their pregnancies and were 100 percent committed to success. They had so little time on a day-to-day basis, that for them to carve out one hour per week for their health was truly an indication of how serious they were. From the start, we dropped all processed grains and flours from their diet. We also eliminated products labeled "fat free" that were actually loaded with sugar and other fillers that over-stimulated the fat storage hormone insulin. The ladies were encouraged to include healthy fats in the form of nuts, natural nut butters, fish oils, cold water fish, flaxseeds, flaxseed oil and olive oil. In addition to helping with weight loss and hormonal balance, the inclusion of omega-3 fats in their diet helped all of them with sluggish digestion (all four had constipation issues off and on). Last but not least, all four women memorized and applied their new mantra at every meal: what is my protein source?

I am thrilled to tell you that as I write this passage, these ladies have been on my program for two months and are all almost at their goal weights. In addition, Elena has had her cholesterol re-tested and it is within normal range. The ladies adhered to the 30 days to re-setting your metabolic code step, and each has optimized her digestion and energy. They still attend meetings with me and are thrilled that their friends and relatives have noticed their new shape. They are down many sizes and are looking and feeling great. Bravo, my fabulous housewives!

part 3

Keeping It Off

9

Emotional Eating

"I don't eat junk foods and I don't think junk thoughts."

Peace Pilgrim (1908-1981),
American peace activist

When you wake up in the morning, does the snugness of your pants determine your mood? Do you find that when you do start to lose weight, you sabotage those results and binge eat until you experience the horrible feeling of "food guilt"? In truth, at a certain level, we are all emotional eaters. Happy, sad, bored, lonely, frustrated or anxious, we eat! However, if you are in a continual pattern of emotional eating and it is holding you back from reaching your weight-loss and health goals, it is time to examine this issue and break this pattern for good.

In practice, I have met many people who have been dieting for 20 years or more. These people are "lifers" when it comes to the weight-loss world. You name a diet or a program that has been on the market, and they have tried it. I have also met weight-loss seekers who are deeply entrenched in the throws of emotional and chaotic eating and cannot seem to get it under control. For example, when taking an initial health history of an individual and recording the times they eat during the day, some people reveal they awake from sleep in the middle of the night and binge eat whatever is in the fridge. Other people have told me that nighttime is what "gets them" in terms of faulty food patterns. In other words, they report eating perfectly during the day, but when night falls and stresses tend to rise, they grab too much of all the wrong foods. The result? In addition to weight gain, emotional eating and food binging often results in feelings of shame, despair and low self-esteem. More often than not, when people gain and lose weight over and over again, there are more than mere food choices underlying the issue.

Food is one of the most intimate and potentially addictive relationships we develop from an early age. If we use food to soothe, numb or for any other emotional purposes, we run the risk of food running *us*. One of the definitions of insanity is doing the same action over and over again and actually expecting a different result. Without taking care of the emotional baggage that may be at the core of your food issues, you will run the risk of being a "lifer" in the weight-loss world. It is far more wise to dive down to an even deeper level to become conscious of the way you are eating and why. Only by doing this will you be in charge of your food choices.

We Eat the Way We Live

I once read a passage that stated, "We eat the way we live." In addition to being addicted to food hormonally and chemically (from eating too many high-glycemic index (GI) carbohydrates), we also tend to create a habitual pattern of turning to food at stressful or uncomfortable times. From a biochemical level, this makes complete sense. If you are feeling sad, moody or low on energy, eating a sugary treat or a starchy food will cause a temporary secretion of "feel-good chemicals" called endorphins in the brain, thereby improving your mood. In addition, we tend to associate being full with being comforted. Unfortunately, this temporary feeling soon goes away and you are left with feelings of guilt and "why did I just eat that?" thoughts. In addition, during times of stress, we do not crave yogurt or a carrot for energy. If we did, the weight-loss issue would not be as out of control as it is. When emotionally eating and binging, we tend to grab fast foods and sugary treats such as cookies, candies, soda and cereal. While eating in a hurried and chaotic manner, portion size flies out the window and instead of eating one cookie, before you know it, a row and even a bag of cookies is gone!

The emotional connection we have with food begins at an early age. When we are children, if we were sad or fell off our bikes and hurt ourselves, what did Mom or Dad do to make us feel better? In addition to a hug or kiss, we were also rewarded with a sweet to soothe our feelings. It is the "Do you have a boo boo? Here is a cookie to make it all better" scenario! Parents also often use food to discipline. I routinely see parents, in an attempt to have a smooth grocery shop, tell their children they may have a cookie, candy or chocolate if they behave while in the grocery cart. I have also met countless parents attempting to potty train their toddler by using M&Ms as a reward for each successful bathroom trip. You can surely see how this sets up an unhealthy relationship with food from an early age. The association can be likened to the old Pavlovian experiment, where when a bell is rung, a dog salivates and is rewarded with food. Eventually when the bell is rung, food or no food, the dog salivates. Food behaviors are no exception. If you are sad and Mommy rewards you with a candy or chocolate, all is fine. However, the next time you get sad and a parent is not there, what is the stimulus you are expecting to take care of and soothe the situation? Sugar or starchy carbohydrates, of course!

As mentioned, on a certain level we are all emotional eaters. Yet, as for any behavior, there are spectrums. When the degree of emotional eating is holding you back from the joys in life and from hitting your target weight, it is time to take some action. How do you know if you are an emotional eater? A few classic behaviors include:

- Trying repetitively but failing to keep weight off
- Feeling frantic and out of control when eating
- Eating frequently when not hungry
- Binge eating large portions of unhealthy food items
- Eating late at night
- Thinking about food often
- Sabotaging good feelings and weight-loss attempts. (For example, after having a good run of eating well and feeling healthy, you start binge eating at night when you are feeling stressed or anxious.)
- Turning to food during times of stress or despair
- Continuing to eat when full
- Feeling guilty following a food binge, (e.g., telling yourself: I will skip a meal tomorrow, exercise more, etc.)
- Sudden, automatic and absent-minded eating
- Strong cravings for specific foods that have nothing to do with physical hunger

The good news is that, as with implementing any change in your life, the 21-day rule to changing a habit (discussed in Chapter 2) applies. With repetition and by following the three steps below, you can finally take back control.

Changing the Pattern

The definition of emotional eating is "consuming large quantities of comfort foods in a response to feelings instead of hunger." In fact, experts estimate that as much as 75 percent of all overeating is caused by emotions. In order to make long-lasting weight-loss changes, it is most effective to take a physical *and* psychological approach. In addition to making more sensible food choices and revving up your metabolic engine, it is also critical to "check in with yourself" to see if you are eating with awareness. In other words, are you aware of the amount of food you are consuming on a daily basis? Are you gobbling up your food at such a frantic pace that you are not even chewing or enjoying the taste and texture? Are you making any of your own food or do you grab everything you eat on the run? In order to shift back to a state of awareness and mindful eating, there are three main steps that you must take.

1. Identify your triggers.
2. Find a replacement behavior.
3. Practice mindful eating.

1. Identify Your Triggers

While I would love to teach you a method of dodging stress and unpleasant feelings for the rest of your life, it is not possible. Life is filled with ups and downs—from major stressors such as loss of a loved one, loss of a job or a divorce, to life's little everyday stresses such as taking care of the kids, being late for a meeting or missing a deadline. Whatever the trigger is, during times of mild, moderate or intense stress, emotional eaters turn to food to numb and deal with their feelings. I call it the "eating more, feeling less" syndrome. This reaction typically has two roots.

1. Emotional baggage from the past and/or present. While some may turn to excessive alcohol, drugs or work, others may turn to food and overeat to deal with stress.
2. In addition to emotional issues, binge eating the wrong foods tends to make your blood sugar bounce around. This results in intense sugar and starchy carbohydrate cravings, fluctuations in mood and energy and the need for more!

In order to stop a food binge in its tracks, it is vital to identify your food triggers. I recently saw a woman named Magdie who was 5 feet 9 inches and weighed 320 pounds. Her weight had ballooned to an enormous number and she felt chronically depressed, fatigued and disappointed with herself. Magdie was an incredibly personable and warm person, but due to her upset with her body, she began cutting herself off from the world by socializing less and less. She had tried to lose weight several times in the past, but each and every attempt had ended with failure, further weight gain and even more negative emotions. In addition to giving her a nutritional overhaul (she was a drive-through queen, eating an abundant amount of fast food and sugary items), we sat down together to identify her triggers. I was amazed to discover that Magdie could instantly name her food trigger and identify why she had such an unhealthy relationship with food.

As it turns out, years back, her world was rocked by her parent's very abusive relationship, which was followed by an ugly divorce. Experiencing feelings of loneliness, abandonment and despair, Magdie turned to food at a very young age to help her cope with her underlying emotions. As the years went by and others began to date and pair off, Magdie's feelings of loneliness intensified, exacerbating her already unhealthy relationship with food. After identifying her triggers and feeling like she had endured enough self-sabotaging behavior—Magdie decided it was time for a real change. I am happy to report that Magdie is on her way to both emotional and physical health. In addition to seeing a counselor, she has lost over 45 pounds on *The Last 15* and is still going!

Identifying your food triggers is the first major component of finally putting an end to emotional eating. By pinpointing the feelings or thought processes behind the trigger, you can finally take steps to deal with your emotions and make peace with them and yourself.

In order to identity your triggers, it is very importanct that you start keeping a food journal. In addition to monitoring the quality and quantity of food you are consuming daily, if you have over-consumed, it is very helpful to record how you were feeling at that time. By doing so, you will soon notice a distinct pattern between your thoughts, feelings and food. If you find that you need assistance uncovering or dealing with your emotional eating and triggers, seek out a counselor or psychologist who is trained and equipped to help.

2. Find a Replacement Behavior

While studying for my undergraduate degree in psychology, I remember one of my professors lecturing on the importance of replacement behaviors. He stressed that for permanent change to take place, a healthy and more suitable replacement behavior had to be followed. For example, when a smoker quits smoking, he needs to implement a positive and realistic behavior such as chewing gum, exercising or drinking water for the new change to become permanent.

In terms of emotional eating, replacement behaviors are equally important. When you feel the frantic urge to eat and are ready to just grab something, stop, take a breath and try one of the following replacement behaviors:

- Go for a walk with a friend.
- Drink lemon water.
- Drink a cup of green tea.
- Write in your food journal about how you are feeling.
- Read a book.
- Call a friend.
- Go for a drive.
- Do housework such as laundry or ironing.

Trust me, replacement behaviors are critical to implementing change. While in the throws of a stressful event, grabbing the cookie is much simpler (and more attractive) than making a cup of tea. However, until the habit is broken, you need to force yourself to engage in an alternate behavior. It is important to take a moment and think about a replacement behavior that is realistic and attractive to you and that can fit into your current lifestyle.

A recent client named Samantha was a self-admitted emotional eater. She was extremely dissatisfied with her career and dreaded going to work at her desk job every day. Due to boredom and a bad case of the blahs, Samantha turned to candy as an instant pick-me-up. Everyday she would snack on licorice, wine gums and chocolate almonds for a quick boost. Eventually, her cravings for these sweet treats were so intense she needed to have them daily to keep her energy up and to calm her nerves.

Unfortunately, due to a sedentary lifestyle, too much high-GI snack food and late night eating, Samantha found that the pounds were starting to add up. Before she realized it, she had 15 extra pounds she was not happy with. In order to effect a permanent change for Samantha, we had to find a replacement behavior that would stick. Samantha was already used to snacking sitting at her desk, so we simply replaced the candy with "free foods" such as sliced cucumbers, cut up broccoli or baby carrots. She also made sure to drink more water and green tea while at the office for its metabolic boosting effects. Instead of brooding over her unsatisfying job each day after work, she decided to join a gym and get more active. Samantha now works out five times a week and is in the process of switching to a new career. She committed to following the 30 days to re-setting her metabolic code and quickly and easily lost the 15 extra pounds. Of course, there is much more to Samantha's story than her weight loss. However, taking charge of her health and food choices and losing the weight were the impetus to take back control of her life. Her improved self confidence and clarity from losing weight and feeling good about herself are "tipping over" into all areas of her life. Remember, when you feel better, you do better. That is the bottom line.

3. Practice Mindful Eating

Do you remember the Simon and Garfunkel song called *Feeling Groovy* that started with the lyrics, "Slow down, you move too fast; you've got to make the morning last?" This line offers great advice: in order to enjoy our short time here on Earth, we need to stop, take notice of our surroundings and enjoy. The same principles apply to eating. In order to really and truly enjoy our food, we need to slow down, take small bites, chew and enjoy the entire flavor. This is what I refer to as mindful eating. Mindful eating is the opposite of emotional eating and involves all five senses on a very intimate and conscious level. Consider the difference.

The Difference between Emotional and Mindful Eating

Emotional Eating	Mindful Eating
Emotional eating is quick and sudden. Within 1–2 minutes, you can gobble up an entire meal and then some without even tasting the real essence of the food!	Mindful eating is slow and gradual. You enjoy and are aware of every element of your food including taste, color, texture and flavor.
Emotional eating is triggered by a certain feeling or situation. For example, your boss has yelled at you or you are in a fight with your boyfriend.	Mindful eating is in response to true signs of hunger.
Emotional eating consists of overeating the wrong types of foods. Symptoms such as bloating and feelings of guilt often accompany the food binge.	Mindful eating never results in feelings of guilt. Following a meal or snack, there is a feeling of being satisfied, not stuffed.
Emotional eating is absent minded and unconscious. For example, you realize you just ate an entire bag of chips—after the fact.	When you eat mindfully, you know exactly how much food you have consumed.

In order to eat with awareness, when you sense the urge to eat, you must stop, take a breath and focus your awareness back to how you are feeling. Is it hunger or is it stress? Try implementing the following steps when starting to practice mindful eating.

- Take sips of water between each bite.
- Do not take the entire bag or container of food. It is best to dish out

the amount or serving size you would like to eat in a small dish or bowl.

- Use your knife, fork and spoon while eating; they will slow you down. Take breaths between bites and chew your food.
- Do not keep high-GI snack foods in the house. If the temptation is there, you will likely give in to it during times of stress.
- Play the "name it" game. While sitting down for a meal, pick one or two things that you are really enjoying about your food. Is it the color of the strawberry? The crunch of the walnut? This will slow down your eating and snap you back into awareness.
- Try to make your meals last a minimum of 20 minutes. It takes 20 minutes for the stretch receptors in your stomach to say to your brain, "Hey! I am full."
- Invest in chewing gum or chewable vitamin C. When you are experiencing the urge to grab and gobble, pop two chewable vitamin Cs in your mouth to slow you down and curb cravings.
- Do not skip meals. Skipping meals will lead to overeating.
- Do not eat until you are uncomfortably full (until your pants feel snug). Eat until you are approximately 80 percent full.
- Allow yourself to get hungry and feel your stomach grumble. It is important to be able to identify real hunger vs. eating merely out of boredom or eating according to the clock.
- Talk to a friend or a trusted family member about the issues you are having with food. There are also wonderful psychologists and counselors who specialize in this field and can be of great value.

"Whoops, I Did It Again"

Uh oh! Here we go again. You have tried implementing the above steps, and presto—during an emotional time, you hit rock bottom and fell smack off the mindful-eating path. Don't panic; all is not lost. And don't waste your energy on food guilt. Simply stand up, brush off your ego and move on. Depending on the root cause of your emotional eating and the length of time you have had an unhealthy relationship with food, it may take some time to take back control of your eating habits. For starters—repetition, repetition, repetition! You need to follow your new practice of awareness eating for a minimum of 21 days for a habit to start to form (30 days is better!). In addition, eating with awareness is an art that has to be mastered. Everyone's dance with food is different; it all depends on your emotional past and present. If you do stray from the weight-loss path during an emotional time and go on a food binge, that is okay. Two steps forward, one step back. Simply continue implementing the three steps above and before long, you will find peace and control with your diet.

Keep in mind that winning the weight-loss battle more often than not involves a psychological component. *The Last 15* would not be a complete weight-loss guide if it did not deal with the psychology of eating and change. Once you take control of the underlying issues, you will feel an enormous burden lifted that will allow you to enjoy food and nutrition without negative emotional results.

Sarah

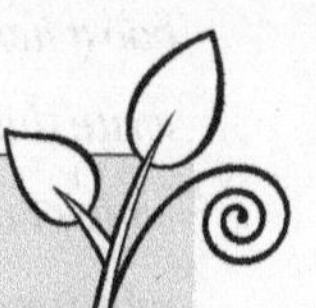

Age: 27

Height: 5 feet 5 inches

Current weight: 152 pounds

Goal weight: 125 pounds

Sarah described her body image and relationship with food as unhealthy and out of control. From an early age, the focus of discussion at Sarah's household was on being overweight and dieting. With both of her parents overweight and Sarah struggling with her weight as a child, Sarah had a distorted relationship with food almost her entire life. In fact, she remembers a nutritionist as early as age eight.

Due to the constant pressure to be thin, Sarah was desperate to gain control over her issues. Unfortunately, the spectrum swung too far and Sarah lost 60 pounds very quickly at age 19; she was diagnosed with an-

orexia nervosa. Due to her extreme calorie restriction, Sarah lost her menstrual cycle for over a year and a half. A couple of years following, she decided to leave home and attend university where her struggle for control swung the other way, causing her to gain 65 pounds.

It was obvious that Sarah had a deeply emotional and unhealthy relationship with food and needed to deal with those emotional issues. Sarah also needed to control her cravings and once again boost her metabolism with the food principles outlined in this book. Her metabolism was extremely sluggish due to her previous up-and-down weight-loss attempts, e.g., she was working out intensely five times a week and was not losing.

Sarah began to keep a food journal to record what she was eating on a daily basis. She also agreed to stock her home with healthy food choices.

She knew if she had candy or cookies in her home, in a time of stress, it would be too easy to reach for them. Sarah was also realistic about her weight-loss goals. She wanted to take off her excess weight in a healthy and hormonally balanced manner that would make her feel in control, boost her confidence and enhance the current relationship she was in. As I write this, Sarah has lost 17 pounds and is thrilled to finally be taking back control of her emotions and food. She is on the road to having a positive relationship with food that she hopes to pass on to her future family.

10

Putting It All Together

"Those who think they have no time for healthy eating will sooner or later have to find time for illness."

Edward Stanley (1799-1869),
English Statesman

When giving seminars across the country, I always ask the following question of my audience: "Please raise your hand if you are not busy, if you have an abundant amount of time in your day and if you are also totally stress free!" Of course, I ask this question in jest. We all live in a world that tends to be go, go, go; we try to fit as much in our day as possible. While recognizing that we are all busier than ever, my goal is to make weight loss and healthy eating second nature and eventually effortless. I have never been a fan of diets that recommend weighing foods or counting calories in the long term. I think weight-loss systems or restrictive dietary behaviors promote short-term results. Let's be honest, shall we? If it isn't easy to do, eventually you will give up and go back to your old ways.

I am an advocate of becoming nutritionally aware by understanding what is in your grocery store. Eating healthy and losing weight does not have to feel like a confusing game of science that is difficult, if not impossible, to understand and implement. Similar to any new behavior or change in your life, *The Last 15* initially takes some focus (and you are focusing already simply by reading this book!). However, before you know it, you will think back to your old ways of unhealthy eating and living and think, "How did I ever get through my day feeling like that?" From CEOs and traveling business people to stay-at-home moms who have three kids—*The Last 15* can be incorporated into even the most confusing and busy schedules.

This chapter is one of the most important of the entire book. Throughout the next few pages, you will learn how to take all that you have learned in previous chapters and easily implement healthy food habits into your life. In other words, I put all the pieces of this puzzle together one last time and present it in quick and easy "short bites" that can make the process crystal clear. From interpreting food labels to eyeballing food amounts and taking the proper supplements, you will soon have all you need to know to make *The Last 15* the last diet you will ever need.

Okay, You Have Reached Your Goal Weight—Now What?

Can you hear that? That is me clapping and standing up to acknowledge the fact that you have hit your goal weight! Bravo, with your focus and determination you have officially joined *The Last 15* club. Now that you have reached your goal and feel great, I want to ensure that you keep the weight off and maintain your incredible results for life.

In order to keep your metabolism revved and assure that you do not start to put weight back on, it is important to sum up the nutritional approaches presented in Part 2—the rest of your life. These principles will allow you to eat delicious food whether at home or on the go without the pounds starting to creep back on. As mentioned, if you have not yet hit your goal weight, you can safely stay on the 30 days to re-setting your metabolic code for as long as it takes , depending on how much weight you need to lose (on average, you will lose 10 to 15 pounds within the first 30 days) and 8-10 pounds or more per month for each month following.

The Last 15 Dietary Approach for Life

- 40–50% of total daily calories from low-glycemic index (GI) carbohydrates such as whole grains, vegetables, fruits and beans
- 25–30% of total daily calories from lean protein sources such as fish, chicken, turkey, soy, eggs, low-fat dairy products and occasional lean beef, if desired
- 25–30% of total daily calories from the "good" fats such as avocados, olive oil, flaxseeds, flaxseed oil, walnuts, almonds, cashews, natural nut butters, sesame seeds, fish and fish oils.

Following your 30 days to re-setting your metabolic code, a typical day on *The Last 15* food program will incorporate on average the following servings per day:

- Grain products: 2–4 servings (150 calories each)
- Vegetables: 5–6 servings (30 calories each)

- Fruits: 2–4 servings (100 calories each)
- Milk products and milk alternatives (low fat): 2 servings (100 calories each)
- Meat and alternatives: 2–3 servings (150 each)

To jam pack your day with high-quality foods filled with anti-oxidants and plant nutrients, you need to eat alive to feel alive. In other words, try to have something colorful and alive (fruits and/or vegetables) at each and every meal or snack.

The Last 15 dinner plate should look like this:

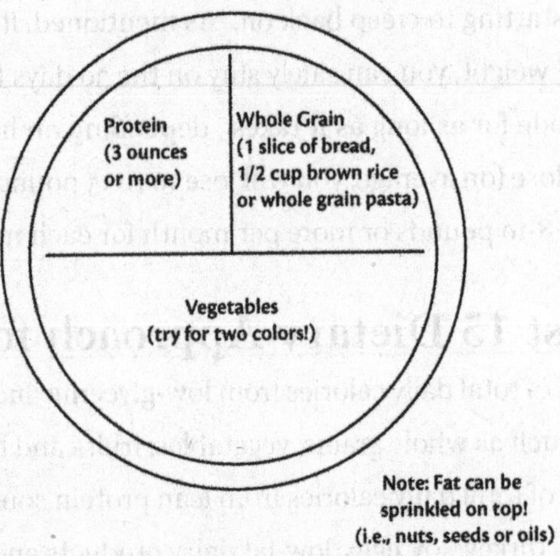

The Last 15 morning protein smoothie should look like this:

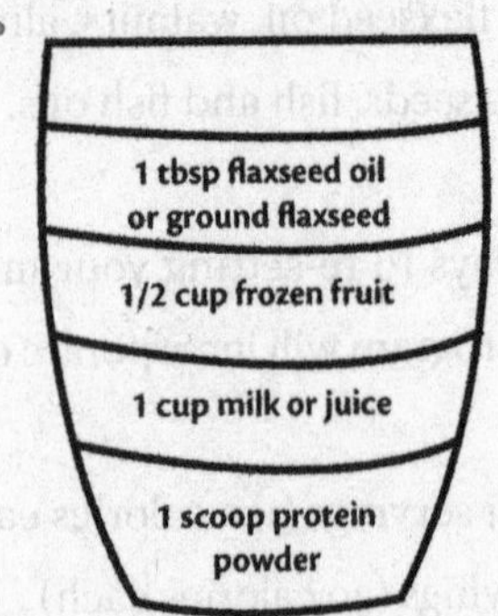

Food Rules

In order to stay in hormonal balance, all the while enjoying and even celebrating with food, follow the food rules below. They will be of great value in helping you stay on track.

Food Rule #1: The 80–20 Rule

In my previous books, I often refer to the 80–20 rule of eating. If you are familiar with this rule, terrific! This approach to eating is so important to maintaining your new svelte figure, it deserves reiteration. The 80–20 of rule of eating states that to maintain your ideal body weight and to preserve an ideal state of health and wellness, you should stick to healthy and delicious eating 80 percent of the time and allow yourself to fall off the health wagon 20 percent of the time—on special occasions, weekends, your birthday, etc. By following this philosophy of eating, you will automatically build in enough flexibility for those times when you do not have as much control over your food intake. Keep in mind that *The Last 15* food is so delicious and filling, you will not feel a sense of deprivation or the urge to cheat. In addition, your food intake is based on achieving hormonal balance that will stop your cravings and the desire to overeat refined flours or other sweets. By following the foods plan outlined in the previous chapters, your palate will shift towards naturally sweet and satisfying alternatives.

The idea of the 80-20 rule of eating allows you to have fun with your food, whether eating healthy or cheating, without feelings of deprivation or restriction. It is designed to help you relax about your food intake at family functions, when traveling, when dining out and the like.

The 80–20 rule of eating can also be applied to certain treats you simply do not want to give up. For example, I recently had a client who told me she could follow the 30 days to re-setting her metabolic code without a problem, but she simply could not (and would not) give up her daily latte with sprinkles of chocolate. Perfect! She identified her barriers and enabled me to create a program that would work around them. She knew that without her latte she would feel that she was being deprived and would be more prone to cheat. I am happy to report that this woman has shed over 30 pounds in a very short time, and yes, she still enjoys her daily latte with chocolate sprinkles!

Food Rule #2: Pick One Day a Week for Light Eating

To optimize digestion and continue with weight-loss success and weight maintenance, I have found it very beneficial to overall health to pick one day out of the week when you eat on the light side. In other words, eat all three meals and one snack, but fill most of your meals with vegetables, fruits and lean proteins. In addition, flush your system with six to eight glasses of water with fresh squeezed lemon. Lemon juice is a natural astringent that will help to clean out the pipes and boost energy. Remember one of the most important mottos of this book: you are only as healthy as your digestive system. It is of the utmost importance that you digest and eliminate properly every day.

Food Rule #3: You Always Have the 30 Days to Re-Setting Your Metabolic Code

Uh oh, it is starting to creep back on! If during a stressful time or a prolonged vacation you lose your healthy eating habits and have not been able to get them back, do not panic. Remember, you are in the know when it comes to nutrition and hormonal balance. If you start to slowly gain five or even 10 pounds and feel out of control, this is the time to go back to the 30 days to re-setting your metabolic code and regain control of your hormones and food cravings. The good news is, you did it once and you can quickly do it again.

If you find yourself gaining a few extra pounds, nip it in the bud. Losing the path to health for a few days or even a week will not cause you to gain back all of the weight you have lost. However, if you continue to make poor choices and your new health patterns become a thing of the past, you will be at risk of falling back into your old faulty eating habits. To avoid this scenario, I highly recommend sharpening your food focus by once again keeping a food journal, re-visiting the 30 days to re-setting your metabolic code and grocery shopping for healthy, grab-and-go basics.

Quality of Life by Choice, Not Chance

"If you don't do what's best for your body, you're the one who comes up on the short end."

—Julius Erving, American basketball player

Similar to learning any new skill, when first learning about nutrition, I am a big advocate of people gathering as much information on the subject as they can. This is what I am referring to with "quality of life by choice, not chance." My goal in writing this book is to provide all the information that you need to know about weight loss, metabolic boosting and nutrition so you can take this information and improve your health and the health of those you love. Part of this knowledge includes being a savvy and informed label reader and grocery shopper. From calories per serving to identifying trans fat in processed foods—it is important to know exactly what you are putting in your body.

Understanding Nutrition Facts Labels

If you have trouble interpreting food labels and find it a confusing game of science, you are certainly not alone. In fact, a recent research study that appeared in *The Journal of Preventative Medicine* showed that a significant amount of people from a variety of educational backgrounds demonstrated deficiencies in understanding food labels. A majority of the confusion was derived from misinterpreting serving sizes and failing to calculate properly. While interpreting Nutrition Facts labels may seem like a daunting task initially, it certainly does not have to be. This skill is very important as it ensures that you buy healthy food for your home and do not get tricked by slick advertising and labeling. Let's clear up the confusion on this matter once and for all, shall we? Follow the explanations below and refer to the sample label for reference.

Nutrition Facts

Serving Size 1 cup (228g)
Servings Per Container 2

Amount Per Serving

Calories 250	Calories from Fat 120
	% Daily Value*
Total Fat 13g	**20%**
Saturated Fat 5g	**25%**
Trans Fat 2g	
Cholesterol 30mg	**10%**
Sodium 660mg	**28%**
Total Carbohydrate 31g	**10%**
Dietary Fiber 0g	**0%**
Sugars 5g	
Protein 5g	

Vitamin A 4%	•	Vitamin C 2%
Calcium 15%	•	Iron 4%

*Percent Daily Values are based on a 2,000 calorie diet. Your Daily Values may be higher or lower depending on your calorie needs:

	Calories:	2,000	2,500
Total Fat	Less than	65g	80g
Sat Fat	Less than	20g	25g
Cholesterol	Less than	300mg	300mg
Sodium	Less than	2,400mg	2,400mg
Total Carbohydrate		300g	375g
Dietary Fiber		25g	30g

Calories per gram:
Fat 9 • Carbohydrate 4 • Protein 4

Serving Size

Serving sizes are located at the top of the label. These amounts are standardized to make comparisons with other food items easier. Serving sizes are provided in familiar units such as cups or grams. Serving size is the most important information to pay attention to. While a food item may appear lower in fat or calories, the serving size of the item might be quite small. In other words, you may eat up to two or even three times the serving size that is listed on the package, hence you are eating two to three times the sugar or calories listed. Food companies are making their serving sizes smaller in order to make their nutritional numbers appear smaller.

Calories (kcal)

A calorie is a unit of energy and differs from food to food. Calories on the Nutrition Facts panel provide a measurement of how much energy you obtain after eating a serving size of a specific food. Watch calories closely. As you already know, labels such as "fat free" or "sugar free" do not necessarily mean the food in question is low in calories.

Nutrients

The next section on the food label refers to total fat, saturated fat, cholesterol, carbohydrates (including fiber and added sugars), protein, vitamin A, C, calcium and iron. Other nutrients may be included if the manufacturer decides to do so. As mentioned, effective January 2006, all labels also have to indicate the presence of trans fatty acids.

Percent Daily Values

Percent daily values provide an estimate of the percentage of a nutrient from one serving in a 2000-calorie diet.

- 5% or less of a nutrient: it's considered a poor source of that nutrient.
- 10–20% of your daily recommended amount of a nutrient: it's a good source of that nutrient.
- More than 20%: it's high in that nutrient.

Total Fat

This refers to the weight of fat (in grams) in one serving of the food.

Saturated Fat

This refers to the weight of saturated fat (in grams) in one serving of the food.

Sodium

This refers to the weight of sodium (in milligrams) in one serving of the food. Daily sodium intake should be less than 2400 mg for a 2000-calorie diet.

Protein

This refers to the weight of protein (in grams) in one serving of the food.

Total Carbohydrates

This refers to the weight of both complex and simple carbohydrates (in grams) in one serving of the food.

Sugars

This refers to the weight of simple carbohydrates (in grams) in one serving of the food; to find out how many complex carbohydrates are in the food subtract sugars from total carbohydrates. Keep in mind that 1 teaspoon of sugar = 4 grams (16 calories).

In general, when you are scanning Nutrition Facts labels, you want to look for foods that are high in fiber, minerals and vitamins and low in sugar, sodium, cholesterol and fats (especially trans fatty acids and saturated fats). Most processed and packaged foods use fats to extend shelf life, coloring to attract the consumer's eye and sugar to enhance taste. As a general rule, the more processed food you remove from your diet, the better!

When eating fresh, whole food such as fruits, vegetables, lean proteins, nuts, seeds and healthy oils, you do not need to worry about food labels; this food is straight from nature's goodness. In general, the less packaged, the better. For a healthier shop, try to stick to the exterior aisles of the grocery store where fruits, vegetables, lean meats, cheeses and eggs are located. Minimize grocery items from the interior aisles, which contain packaged, processed and refined goods.

Understanding the Ingredients List

In addition to the Nutrition Facts panel, the ingredients list is also a very important piece of information. Ingredients are listed in order of most to least by weight. Beware of foods that start out with the first one to two ingredients from sugar (high fructose corn syrup, sucrose), fats and oils (vegetable oils, soybean oil) or salt. If these ingredients appear early on in the list, it is likely not a healthy choice. In addition, as a general rule, the shorter the ingredients list, the better the choice. For the most part, you should be able to pronounce and understand everything that is listed!

In addition to food labels, certain food items also have permission to use specific terms that are regulated and are uniform, ensuring that no matter what food or product they describe, they always mean the same thing. These terms are regulated according to specific criteria by the Food and Drug Administration (FDA). Here are definitions of the most frequently used terms:

- Fat free = 0.5 grams of fat or less
- Calorie free = 5 calories or less
- Sugar free = 0.5 grams of sugar or less
- Sodium free = 5 mg of sodium or less
- Cholesterol free = 2 mg of cholesterol or less
- Low fat = 3 grams of fat or less
- Low in saturated fat = 1 gram of saturated fat or less
- Low cholesterol = 20 mg of cholesterol or less
- Low sodium = 140 mg of sodium or less
- Very low sodium = 35 mg of sodium or less
- Low calorie = 40 calories or less
- Reduced calorie = at least 25% less energy (calories) than a comparable product
- High = 20% or more of daily value
- Good = 10 to 19% of daily value
- Good source of fiber = 4 grams or more of fiber

Note: For a list of food additives, preservatives and colors that you should avoid, please refer to the appendix.

Eyeballing Your Food Portions

In addition to becoming an informed label reader, I am also a fan of people being able to eyeball their food portions. In North America, we tend to suffer from an affliction I call "portion distortion disorder." In other words, we tend to eat more than we realize. Consider the following facts.

- The average size of a bagel has nearly doubled since the 1980s.
- Most convenience stores boast a drink container that holds a whopping 64 ounces of fluid.
- Many fast food chains offer "value meals," where it is more economical to pay less for more food.
- The standard dinner plate used in most restaurants has increased from 10 to 12 inches.
- According to the U.S. Department of Agriculture, the average American diet has increased from 1,854 calories to 2,002 calories in the last 2 decades (source: American Institute for Cancer Research)
- In the 1950s, a hamburger patty was approximately 1.6 to 2 ounces. Now, it can be as large as 8 ounces!
- A recent study at the University of North Carolina showed that since 1977, hamburgers have increased nearly 23 percent, with 97 more calories. French fries have grown by 16 percent, and soft drinks by 52 percent.

Due to the ever-changing quantity of food we purchase and serve, people have lost touch with what is an appropriate amount to eat. Instead of eating until we are satisfied, we tend to overeat until we are bloated and our pants actually feel too tight! You all know the feeling. When you over-consume by eating too much of the wrong foods you can instantly feel a significant drop in energy as you enter a "food coma." In addition, when you overeat (which typically occurs later in the evening) it is not uncommon to feel the side effects the next day. Physically and mentally, eating too many sugars, refined flours, fats and calories can result in a "food hangover" that lasts for anywhere from 24 to 48 hours, depending on your digestive capacity.

Paying attention to portion size, both in and outside of your home, is a critical tool to understanding what a normal portion size is. Keep in mind that research clearly identifies that people will eat what they are served or what is on their plate, whether hungry or not. The result? Excess calories and excess weight.

Here are a few key measurements to be aware of:

- 1 gram of fat = 9 calories.
- 1 gram of protein = 4 calories.
- 1 gram of carbohydrate = 4 calories.
- 4 grams of sugar = 1 teaspoon of sugar

Here are some tips to help you properly eyeball your food portions.

- 1 fruit serving = ½ cup canned or 1 medium fruit (about the size of a tennis ball)
- 1 meat, poultry or fish serving = 3 oz. (about the size of a deck of cards)
- 1 dairy serving = 8 oz. (the size of a container of individual yogurt)
- 1 grain = 1 slice bread, pre-sliced (about the size of a cassette tape), or ½ cup pasta (about the size of an adult woman's palm, stacked 1 inch high)
- 1 vegetable serving = ½ cup cooked or canned vegetables (about ½ a baseball)
- 1 fat serving = 1 teaspoon (about the size of four stacked dimes)

What about Supplements?

Recently, I had a gentleman visit my office and bring in all of his daily supplements. This kind man was slightly type A with his approach to health and wellness, and he described himself as a "health nut." When I asked him what supplements he was taking, the list went on and on! In fact, I counted out his daily supplement regime and it turned out he was taking 46 pills and capsules each day!

I must come clean: I am a big foodie. In other words, I like people to get a majority of their nutrition from high-quality food sources. Yet, even with a perfect diet, which few of us have, I think using supplements as a nutritional safety net and as a natural insurance policy is very important. From lack of sunshine to stress to poor soil quality and faulty food choices—supplements can fill in the gaps for health. What should you take daily? Here are a few supplements that are core to overall health and wellness.

High-Quality Multi-Vitamin

To bridge any dietary gaps, a daily multi-vitamin is recommended. In fact the American Medical Association announced their new position that all adults should take a daily multi-vitamin with minerals to help prevent chronic disease. Supplementing with a daily multi-vitamin has been shown to improve the grades, behavior and focus in school for children and teenagers.

When selecting a multi-vitamin, many people ask me about the difference between RDA (Recommended Daily Allowance) and ODA (Optimal Daily Allowance). RDAs were instituted over 40 years ago by the U.S. Food and Nutrition Board as a standard for the daily amounts of vitamins needed by a healthy person. Unfortunately, the amounts they recommended gave the bare minimum required to ward off deficiency diseases such as beriberi, rickets, scurvy and night blindness. I always refer to the fact that in my practice as a nutritionist, I have never seen one person with a deficiency syndrome such as scurvy (lack of vitamin C) or rickets (lack of vitamin D). I have, however, seen many individuals with what I refer to as "gluttony syndromes" or "faulty food syndromes" such as heart disease, high cholesterol, obesity, stroke and a variety of cancers. The RDA recommendations, unfortunately, do not address the amounts needed to maintain maximum health; they take a borderline health approach.

The ODA recommendations represent new levels designed for optimal health (not simply the absence of disease) that go beyond those of the RDA. Science has shown the ODA levels to have disease-preventing effects and to be perfectly safe. I recommend following these as there is no reason to exceed the ODA levels, unless recommended by your doctor. See the appendix for an RDA vs. ODA chart.

Multi-vitamins are now designed to fit individual health needs. You will find there are specific multi-vitamins for athletes, children, weight loss, heart health, anti-aging and even skin! It is important to take your multivitamin with food to properly absorb the fat soluble vitamins, A, D, E and K. It is also important to purchase a supplement that contains no artificial colors, sweeteners, preservatives or flavors. Please refer to the Product Recommendation list in the appendix for suggested supplements.

Distilled Fish Oil Supplement

Do you remember when your grandmother or mother used to force you to take a spoonful of cod liver oil? Well, if you have ever tried that once, I assure you, you will never want to try it again! Luckily, we have come a long way when it comes to fish oil supplements: they are now available in capsule and flavored form. You will recall from Chapter 8 on healthy fats that getting enough omega-3 into the diet can have enormous health benefits for your skin, hair, heart and overall immune system function.

Research has shown that omega-3 fats are beneficial for weight loss and help you to burn more fat. In a study published in *The International Journal of Obesity*, researchers found that those taking fish oil supplements increased the number of calories they burn in a single day. In the study, two groups were fed exactly the same diet, and one group supplemented with 6 grams of fat in the form of butter, olive oil, sunflower oil and peanut oil, while the other group supplemented with 6 grams of fish oil. The total intake of omega-3 fats was 1.8 grams per day. The table below highlights the changes in fat oxidation, metabolic rate and body fat after only three weeks.

Effects of Dietary Fish Oil on Body Fat Mass

	With fish oil	**Without fish oil**
Measurement of body fat	2 pounds lost	0.7 pounds lost
Daily metabolic rate	1775 calories burned	1710 calories burned

These results show that the group that was supplementing with fish oil burned about 1.1 milligrams of fat per kilo per minute. This is roughly 26 percent higher than the other group who weren't supplementing with fish oil. One of the key reasons for their weight-loss success appears to be that insulin levels were approximately 50 percent lower for those supplementing with fish oils.

In another recent Australian study, researchers found that supplementing with fish oils can assist with weight loss when combined with moderate exercise. Even though dietary intake was exactly the same, overweight individuals who took fish oil supplements and exercised lost an average of 2 kg (4.5 lbs) over three months, unlike the groups that took sunflower oil and exercised (sunflower oil does not contain omega-3 fat). Overweight individuals who exercised and took sunflower oil did not lose any weight. The researchers believe that fish oil increases the fat-burning ability of the body by improving the blood flow to muscles during exercise.

As you have learned throughout this book, hormonal balance is of the utmost importance for weight loss and is one of the primary foundations of *The Last 15*. A balanced diet that includes plenty of omega-3 fatty acids from fish oils is one of the main components to achieving and maintaining hormonal balance.

Due to the fact that most North Americans are critically low in omega-3 fats and too high in omega-6 fats (creating the perfect environment for inflammation), I highly recommend a fish oil supplement of 1 to 2 grams daily for weight loss and as one of the core elements of any supplement program. When selecting fish oil supplements, it is important to purchase one that is distilled and free from toxicity. In addition, it is best to select fish oil that is made from smaller fish such as sardines and anchovies (see the Product Resource list). The smaller the fish, the shorter the lifespan and, consequently, the lower the accumulation of toxicity. Store your fish oil supplements in the refrigerator. Be sure to talk to your doctor prior to supplementing with omega-3 fats if you are on a blood thinner medication or going for surgery.

Protein Powder for Your Morning Smoothies

Remember, protein foods are not as quickly obtained as carbohydrates. Because of this, it is important to have easy-to-eat protein options on hand. Keeping a chocolate or vanilla whey isolate protein powder on hand for your daily breakfast smoothie or a snack at the office makes it easy to get your protein intake during the morning rush.

Probiotics—the Friendly Bacteria

Probiotics are dietary supplements that contain strains of bacteria that can help to replenish proper bacterial microflora and can fight off unwanted bacteria such as E.coli. There are many strains of probiotics, with the most common type being Lactobacilli and Bifidobacteria. Probiotics have been shown to have the following benefits on overall health:

- Lower cholesterol levels
- Clear yeast from the body, e.g., systemic yeast or yeast infections
- Improve irritable bowel syndrome
- Improve overall digestive health (i.e. constipation, bloating etc.)
- Alleviate allergic responses
- Decrease inflammatory response
- Produce many important enzymes and vitamins such as Vitamin B, Vitamin K, lactase, fatty acids and calcium
- Improve the immune system's overall functioning

As you already know, if your digestion is not optimal and you are not absorbing and eliminating properly, achieving your health goals (weight loss or other) is extremely difficult. I am an advocate of taking a baseline of probiotics daily as a nutritional safety net to a healthy digestive system. In addition, supplementing with probiotics following antibiotic therapy is very important for avoiding the overgrowth of yeast in the body. While antibiotics may be necessary to eliminate an infectious agent, they unfortunately wipe out the "good" and the "bad" bacteria. It is important to restore proper digestive balance with a probiotic.

When consumers first seek a probiotic supplement, the choices can seem overwhelming. When selecting a brand, keep the following tips in mind:

1. Select a mixed strain probiotic. Probiotics are available in several strains that have different effects on the body. Using a combination of probiotics (that contains both Lactobacillus acidophilus for the small intestine and Bifidobacterium bifidum for the large intestine) is the best way to go.

2. Each capsule should contain a minimum of 1 billion organisms per capsule. I know this may sound like an extremely high number, but remember, we are talking about bacteria!
3. Purchase a probiotic that needs to be kept in the refrigerator.

What about Yogurt?

Several yogurts on the market now advertise having a probiotic content. According to the Food and Drug Administration (FDA), in order for a refrigerated product to be called "yogurt," it must be produced by culturing permitted dairy ingredients with a bacterial culture, which contains *Lactobacillus bulgaricus* and *Streptococcus thermophilus.* In addition, the National Yogurt Association developed its own seal to identify viable culture in a yogurt called "Live & Active Culture" seal. In order for manufacturers to carry the seal, refrigerated yogurt products must contain at least 100 million cultures per gram at the time of manufacturing.

While I think yogurt is a wonderful addition to any diet and does contain a certain amount of viable friendly bacteria, for therapeutic reasons, it is best to add a supplement to your daily regime.

Note: The above is a baseline supplement regime. Sometimes supplementation with specific nutrients may be appropriate in order to address individual specific needs. For example, CoQ10 may be recommended for those at risk of heart disease. For one-on-one supplement recommendations for specific conditions, please consult your doctor or your primary natural health care practitioner.

What about Exercise?

"You have to stay in shape. My grandmother, she started walking five miles a day when she was 60. She's 97 today and we don't know where the hell she is."

—Ellen Degeneres

No weight-loss regime or healthy lifestyle would be complete without the addition of exercise. To complete the picture of health, exercise is an equally important insurance policy that has enormous benefits. Similar to eating thermogenic foods that boost metabolism and drinking plenty of water, exercise is a fundamental component that helps you flex that metabolic engine and shed excess weight. Keep in mind that our muscles are very needy. In fact, for every pound of muscle you carry, your body requires and burns 50 more calories per day to sustain it. In addition, regular exercise increases circulation, improves heart health, increases endurance and lowers stress. What could be better? Regular exercise also:

- Reduces the risk of premature death
- Reduces the risk of developing and/or dying from heart disease
- Reduces high blood pressure or the risk of developing high blood pressure
- Reduces high cholesterol or the risk of developing high cholesterol
- Reduces the risk of developing colon cancer and breast cancer
- Reduces the risk of developing diabetes
- Reduces or maintains body weight
- Builds and maintains healthy muscles, bones and joints
- Reduces depression and anxiety
- Improves psychological well-being
- Enhances work, recreation and sport performance
- Promotes rhythmic deep breathing
- Improves self-confidence
- Improves quality of sleep
- Increases mental focus
- Improves body shape
- Tones musculature
- Optimizes digestive capacity
- Improves range of motion of joints

This list is just the tip of the iceberg when it comes to the benefits of exercise. Yet, why is it that so many people find implementing this necessary part of health so difficult? The answer is simple: scheduling and habit. When I broach the subject of exercise with my clients, I am often faced with a familiar response: "I just can't find the time in my day."

We are all so busy with kids, work, and "life stuff." Fitting one extra little thing into your schedule may feel like your delicate house of cards will topple over. In truth, all it takes is a little extra focus, some re-scheduling and commitment. I am currently seeing a mother of five children all under the age of eight—and she home schools! If she can find the time, so can all of us. You must (and I mean *must*) commit to fitting in a minimum of 30 minutes of exercise three times per week. Five times per week or more is optimal and is a goal I recommend aiming for. If you have not exercised in a long time, there is no problem in starting off slowly and building up to it. Because a little pain or discomfort is normal when first starting out, take it easy and build your routine over time. Going too hard and too fast initially can result in an injury that will halt your new and well-intentioned exercise plans.

When I first start to help a client implement exercise into her weekly health regime, I am typically faced with two common questions:

Question: What time of the day should I work out?

Answer: You should work out at the time that works best for you! If you know that you can only fit a workout in by waking up one-half hour earlier, then that is the best time for you. Alternatively, if you can sneak an hour during the day from work or when the kids are in school, by all means go for it!

Question: What type of exercise should I do?

Answer: There are a few components of exercising that are important for a variety of health reasons. They are:

- **Aerobic exercise** (cardiovascular exercises) This type of exercise moves large muscle groups and causes your lungs to breathe more deeply and your heart to work harder to pump blood. Examples include walking, jogging, running, cycling, rowing, swimming, skiing, etc.
- **Weight-bearing exercise** This type of exercise works against the force of gravity. Weight-bearing exercise stimulates the production of bone-building cells called osteoblasts and is critical in the prevention of diseases of bone loss such as osteoporosis. Examples include climbing stairs, dancing, weight training, walking and jogging.
- **Weight training** This type of exercise builds strength and muscles and quickly tones the body. Lifting weights, doing push-ups and pull ups are examples of weight training.
- **Stretching** Pre- and post-workout stretching of the upper and lower body is extremely important to avoid injury and maintain flexibility. I hear too many people complain of chronic stiffness as they get older. This does not have to be the case. However, you need to stretch on a daily basis to improve flexibility and feel the results. Along with drinking a lot of water and getting enough omega-3 fats into your diet, stretching can dramatically and quickly affect the way you feel. Instead of waking up stiff and tight, you will notice you feel noticeably more limber and spry in a short time.

A comprehensive and complete exercise program combines aerobic and weight-bearing exercises such as walking and/or jogging with weights. In addition, core strength exercises such as Pilates and expansive movements such as yoga (Hatha, Ashtanga or other types) provide enormous benefits to flexibility, posture and digestion.

When exercising, monitor your heart rate to ensure you are working hard enough, while not overworking. To measure your resting heart rate, simply count your pulse for 15 seconds and multiply by four (for one minute). When beginning an exercise program, your target heart rate will likely be lower (about 60 percent of your target zone). As your heart rate improves and you exercise harder, your target heart rate can improve to approximately 85 percent of your target zone. Please see the graph below to calculate your target heart rate.

Target Heart Rates According to Age

Age	Target Heart Rate Zone 50–85 %	Average Maximum Heart Rate 100 %
20 years	100–170 beats per minute	200 beats per minute
25 years	98–166 beats per minute	195 beats per minute
30 years	95–162 beats per minute	190 beats per minute
35 years	93–157 beats per minute	185 beats per minute
40 years	90–153 beats per minute	180 beats per minute
45 years	88–149 beats per minute	175 beats per minute
50 years	85–145 beats per minute	170 beats per minute
55 years	83–140 beats per minute	165 beats per minute
60 years	80–136 beats per minute	160 beats per minute
65 years	78–132 beats per minute	155 beats per minute
70 years	75–128 beats per minute	150 beats per minute

Source: *www.americanheart.org*

Your maximum heart rate is about 220 minus your age. The figures in the table are averages, so use them as general guidelines.

Note: Certain blood pressure medication may lower the maximum heart rate, thereby affecting your target heart zone. If you are on such medications, talk to your doctor to find out your target heart rate.

In order to fit exercise into your schedule, take a moment to assess what you think will work for your schedule and lifestyle. The time of year also has a huge impact on what types of exercise you choose. In short, the best type of exercise for you is the one that you will actually find the time to do. Here are some tips to help you make exercise a life-long habit.

- Invest in some home weights (5 and 10 pounds) and do an upper body workout while watching your favorite TV show at night. Isn't it funny? We always seem to find the time for TV!

- Wake up 20 to 30 minutes earlier and start your day off with stretches and a brisk walk. If you are fortunate enough to own a piece of exercise equipment (a bike, treadmill or elliptical machine), make sure you are on it for a minimum of 30 minutes, three times a week.
- Join a fitness club. This does not have to be an expensive venture and allows you to have healthy "me" time for a minimum of three times a week. From classes and equipment to getting a detailed and personalized plan drawn up by a personal trainer—it is definitely worth the time and financial investment. In addition, the cost of joining a health club also gives people an incentive to exercise regularly.
- Use exercise tapes. When my son was born, I invested in a yoga tape, which I used at least three times a week while he was napping. This allowed me the luxury of flexibility in terms of schedule and also ensured I fit it exercise into my new schedule.
- Walk out your front door! I cannot tell you how many successful clients I have seen who simply followed the food principles of *The Last 15*, opened their front door and started walking. It is that simple.
- Schedule exercise appointments as you would any other appointment and stick to them!.
- Monitor your progress so you can see improvements in your strength and endurance, e.g., run five minutes longer than you did the week before and so on.
- Develop an exercise fund, where you save a little extra money for your health. You can invest in yoga classes, a piece of home equipment, high-quality running shoes or a new yoga mat.
- Exercise with a buddy. Having someone to exercise with will hold you more accountable and is more fun!
- You can also get exercise in "spits and spats" throughout your day. Sneaking in some extra calorie-burning exercise will help you maintain the constant positive pressure and flexion necessary to drive up your metabolic engine. Here are some tips.

- Always take the stairs for that extra boost.
- Lunge, baby, lunge! Whether it is lunging across your living room or your nearest park, lunging is an excellent way to tone buttocks and hamstring areas. To perform a lunge, stand with your feet shoulder-width apart, and then step forward, landing with the heel first. Continue the motion until the back knee is nearly touching the ground. Then return to the starting position by driving upward with the front leg. Repeat the exercise by stepping forward with the other leg.
- If possible, walk or ride your bike to work.
- Do your housework at a very fast pace.
- For some extra toning, contract your buttocks musculature while driving.
- If working at a desk job, make sure to get up at least once an hour for a mini walk and stretch.

The Magic Bullet Is You!

"To eat is a necessity, but to eat intelligently is an art."

—La Rochefoucauld (1613-1680, French Duke)

When dieting, a quick fix is one of the key factors that inevitably leads to failure. As you have learned, extreme caloric restriction, or dropping all carbohydrates, does result in temporary weight loss, but it is unhealthy and leads to more weight gain in the future. However, now that you have completed reading *The Last 15*, you have everything you need to ensure lifelong weight-loss success, health and energy.

With that, dear readers, we have reached the end of *The Last 15*. I hope that the information you have acquired over the course of this book will inspire you to take charge and lose those excess pounds permanently. In addition to providing all you need to know about nutrition and weight loss, my other goal in writing this book was to motivate you to take action. In other words, this is not the place for a Jacuzzi experience—that temporary bubbly, good feeling that will wear off soon after you have finished reading. Once you implement these changes in your life for 21 days or more, creating an imprinted, long-term and sustainable habit, you will improve your health and wellness for life.

I once had a doctor friend say to me, "Your genes are not your destiny." What did he mean? He was referring to the fact that even though we all land here on the planet with our own personal genetic history, most of us can have a powerful influence over the state of our health and vitality. The major killers of our time—heart disease, cancer, obesity, type 2 diabetes, high cholesterol and stroke—are all influenced by diet, nutrition, supplements, attitude, belief systems and stress levels. As for weight loss, there is a magic bullet that works—and it is you! Take this information and use it to reach your ultimate potential in health and vitality. Remember one of my key mantras: "When you feel better, you do better. Period." Of course, there is much more to life than the food on your plate, but the quality and quantity of your food choices are the tipping point of health that can add or rob precious years from your life. It is up to you.

You now have all the nutritional tools to put all the pieces of the health puzzle together and make it a rich, joyful and inspiring experience for you and your entire family. Remember, there is no plan B! The road to health and wellness begins and continues with you. In the Recipes section you'll find all you need to experiment with new foods. Use the food journal in the Appendix to track what you are eating on a daily basis, and keep track of your progress with the helpful scales and measurements that guide you through your weight-loss journey. I applaud you for taking charge and implementing positive health changes in your life. Unlike the other chapters, I will not end this one with a success story from one of my clients. Why? I am waiting for yours! I look forward to hearing from you at www.drjoey.com.

Wishing you best health and happiness and a lot of fun along the way.

~Dr. Joey Shulman

11

The Last 15 Recipes

"Take care of your body with steadfast fidelity.
The soul must see through these eyes alone,
and if they are dim, the whole world is clouded."

Johann Wolfgang Von Goethe (1749–1832)
German poet, dramatist, novelist

All of the recipes in this section contain the right proportions of protein, low-glycemic index (GI) carbohydrates and essential fat options to ensure your body is hormonally balanced. Following the 30 days to re-setting your metabolic code, these recipes will help you keep your weight down and your energy up. During the first 30 days, please refer to the sample menus outlined in Chapter 4. If you are following the 30 days to re-setting your metabolic code and find a recipe in the following pages you may enjoy, please keep the following in mind:

- The amount of fruit per recipe. In the first 30 days, two servings of fruit are recommended per day. If you eat more than two servings of fruit, I recommend dropping your grain selection at lunch or using the extra fruit as one of your treats that week.
- If you find a sandwich recipe you would enjoy during the first 30 days, simply drop one of the slices of bread and turn the recipe into an open-faced sandwich.
- During the first 30 days, dinners should contain protein and vegetables only—no grain.

The recipes in the following pages are all well balanced and will keep you satiated in a healthy, weight-conscious and hormonally balanced manner. Please note the serving size at the end of each recipe in case you need to adjust the quantity. Recipes are designed to serve one, two, four or six.

In addition and more importantly, all of the recipes outlined in the following pages taste absolutely delicious! My husband, affectionately deemed "the short-cut chef," has created several recipes with your busy schedule in mind. There are numerous fast and easy options that you can make as you go or prepare in advance and freeze for healthy grab-and-go meals.

In our household, we are big advocates of using fresh herbs, vegetables and fruits.

Please refer to page 256 to see the top five herbs and seasonings to stock in your kitchen on a regular basis.

Bon appetite!

Breakfasts

Breakfast Options

Chocolate Lover's Smoothie

As a devoted chocolate lover, I need to get my chocolate fix on a regular basis. This smoothie recipe satisfies my weakness for chocolate, all the while providing filling protein and essential fats.

Ingredients

soy milk or low-fat milk	1 cup
chocolate protein powder	1 scoop
medium banana, frozen	½
ground flaxseeds or flaxseed oil	1 tsp.
chocolate syrup	1 tsp.

Directions

Simply combine all of the ingredients in the blender, blend on high for 1 minute and enjoy! Serves 1.

Blueberry Banana Smoothie

As an alternative to protein powder, you can fill your morning smoothie with some non-fat yogurt to boost your protein intake. For anti-oxidant and health benefits, blueberries are also a wonderful addition to your morning smoothie. According to the U.S. Department of Agriculture Analyses, blueberries have 40 percent more antioxidant capacity than strawberries. They are also high in vitamin C and can help strengthen the immune system.

Ingredients

medium banana, frozen	½
blueberries, fresh or frozen	½ cup
non-fat vanilla yogurt	¼ cup
skim milk or soymilk	1 cup
pinch of cinnamon	

Directions

Combine all of the ingredients in a blender and purée until smooth. Enjoy! Serves 1.

Anti-Oxidant Blast

Raspberries, blueberries and strawberries are all low-glycemic index (GI) foods and filled with an abundant amount of disease-fighting anti-oxidants called flavonoids, which give these beautiful berries their purple and red hue. In addition to providing the body with an abundant amount of nutrition and goodness, berries also help satisfy your sweet tooth without fluctuating blood sugar levels.

Ingredients

orange juice	1 cup
mixed berries, frozen	¼ cup
mangos, frozen	¼ cup
flaxseed oil	1 tsp.
vanilla protein powder	1 scoop

Directions

Combine all of the ingredients in a blender, purée until smooth and enjoy! Serves 1.

Mocha Protein Shake

For coffee lovers, you can now have the benefit of enjoying your morning java and protein smoothie all in one. While I do not recommend having this shake option daily, it is the perfect creamy and delicious morning treat on weekends. Filled with protein powder and a little bit of flaxseed oil, it will fill you up and keep you fueled.

Ingredients

coffee or herbal coffee substitute, brewed	½ cup
organic frozen yogurt, low-fat or non-fat	½ cup
chocolate protein powder	1 scoop
ice cubes	2–4
flaxseed oil	1 tsp.

Directions

Combine all of the ingredients in a blender, purée until smooth and enjoy! Serves 1.

Vanilla Cream Smoothie

Not everyone is a chocolate lover. Instead of indulging in high-GI vanilla cakes or cupcakes, this vanilla cream smoothie will fill you up, tempt your taste buds and maintain your hormonal balance all at the same time! What could be better?

Ingredients

soy or organic skim milk	1 cup
flaxseed oil	1 tsp.
frozen banana	½
pure vanilla extract	2 tsp.
vanilla protein powder	1 scoop
cinnamon to taste	

Directions

Combine all of the ingredients in a blender, purée until smooth and enjoy! Serves 1.

Blueberry Banana Crunch

The morning is typically the time of day when we tend to be rushing. This is why having a breakfast idea that is quick and easy is of the utmost importance. Keep in mind that you must eat breakfast in order to lose weight and stabilize your blood sugar. If you are looking for a variation to your morning protein shake, try this delicious bowl of goodness.

Ingredients

plain yogurt	½ cup
fresh blueberries	½ cup
banana, sliced	½
All Bran cereal or whole-grain Cheerios	½ cup

Directions

Combine all ingredients in a bowl and enjoy! Serves 1.

Decadent Breakfast Delight

This decadent breakfast may sound too good to be true, but with its protein content and essential fats, it will keep your energy up and your weight down. In addition to being delicious and sweet, dark chocolate is also filled with anti-oxidants that have been shown to benefit heart health.

Ingredients

plain yogurt	1 cup
medium banana, sliced	½
walnuts	10
dark chocolate Cadbury thin bar (100 calories), broken up	1

Directions

Combine all ingredients in a bowl. Break up chocolate and sprinkle over top and enjoy! Serves 1.

Cottage Cheese Crunch

Cottage cheese is an excellent grab-and-go option to stock in your refrigerator. Low in calories and fat and high in protein (120 grams offers 99 calories, 16 grams of protein, 1.2 grams of fat and 6.0 grams of carbohydrates), cottage cheese will keep you filled up, all the while offering a creamy, delicious meal.

Ingredients

low-fat or 1 percent cottage cheese	½ cup
Kashi cereal (high in protein)	½ cup
sliced strawberries	½ cup

Directions

Combine all ingredients in a bowl and enjoy. Serves 1.

Spanish Egg White Omelet

This quick and easy breakfast omelet offers great taste and the perfect combination of protein, carbohydrates and fats. Using one whole egg in the mixture mixed with egg whites offers a greater taste and texture and will prevent the mixture from sticking in the pan.

Ingredients

Omega-3 egg	1
egg whites	8-oz carton
red pepper, diced	3 tbsp
white onion, diced	¼ cup
crimini mushrooms, sliced	¼ cup
salt	½ tsp
black pepper	¼ tsp
minced garlic	½ tsp
olive oil	1 tbsp.
tomato slices	6

Directions

Mix whole egg with egg whites and beat until thoroughly mixed. In non-stick pan, heat oil and add red pepper, white onion, mushrooms and minced garlic. Sautée for 4 to 5 minutes until tender. Add egg mixture, salt, pepper and stir while cooking over medium-high heat. Once egg mixture is fully cooked, divide between two plates. Garnish with tomato slices. Serves 2.

Lunches

Lunch Options

Salmon Caesar Salad

When it comes to salmon, it is always best to go for wild options rather than farmed. The good news is most canned salmon is derived from wild sources and is available in all grocery stores. Salmon is an excellent way to boost your intake of omega-3 fatty acids and is a wonderful protein source.

Ingredients

salmon fillet (wild)	5 oz.
Stonemill sprouted grain bread, toasted	1 piece
romaine or head lettuce	½
low-fat Caesar dressing	1 tsp.
butter	½ tsp.
garlic powder	⅛ tsp.
dill seeds	½ tsp.
salt and pepper to taste	

Directions

Lightly butter Stonemill sprouted grain bread and sprinkle with garlic powder. Bake in oven at 375° F until golden brown. Let bread cool and cut into small pieces for croutons.

Grease baking sheet and place salmon on it. Sprinkle salmon with salt and pepper and squeeze lemon over top. Sprinkle dills seeds on salmon with ½ tsp. of butter over fillet. Broil in oven for 10 to 12 minutes. Combine with lettuce, croutons and dressing and toss sliced salmon in ½ inch slices, place on top salad and serve. Serves 1.

Crispy Tofu Green Bean Salad

This recipe can be made ahead of time and can be stored in the fridge as the perfect grab-and-go lunch at work or at home.

Ingredients

Salad

extra-firm tofu	15 oz.
extra virgin olive oil	1 tsp.
whole-grain pasta, spiral	1 cup
green beans	1 cup
cherry tomatoes, halved	1 cup
fresh dill	1 tbsp.

Dressing

red wine vinegar	2 tbsp.
lemon juice	1 tbsp.
extra virgin olive oil	1 tbsp.
low-sodium soy sauce	1 tsp.
sugar	¼ tsp.
salt	¼ tsp.
black pepper	¼ tsp.
garlic cloves, crushed	½ tsp.

Directions

Cut tofu into 2-inch cubes. Heat 1 tsp. of olive oil in a large nonstick skillet over medium-high heat. Add tofu; sauté 5 minutes, browning on all sides. Remove from pan and allow to cool for 30 minutes.

Meanwhile, cook pasta in boiling water for 4 minutes; add beans, and cook an additional 4 minutes. Drain and rinse with cold water. Combine tofu, pasta mixture, tomatoes and dill in a large bowl.

To prepare dressing, combine vinegar and remaining ingredients in a jar; cover tightly and shake vigorously. Pour dressing over salad; toss well to coat. Cover and refrigerate for 30 minutes. Serves 4.

Mini-Quiche to Go

Quiche is a luncheon or dinner favorite that provides a great source of protein. In order to reduce the fat content, ½ of the mixture should be made with egg whites. Variations of this recipe can be created with the addition of vegetables, different low fat cheeses and spices. The great advantage of this recipe is that you can prepare several in advance and freeze for quick, convenient lunches or last-minute dinners.

Ingredients	
eggs	6
egg whites	16 oz.
low fat Mozzarella cheese, shredded	6 oz.
white onion, diced	½ cup
red pepper,diced	½ cup
fresh cilantro, chopped	¼ cup
broccoli flowerets	½ cup
green olives, sliced	¼ cup
salt	½ tsp.
pepper	¼ tsp.

Directions

Break the eggs into a mixing bowl. Add egg whites and beat until smooth. Add diced onion, red pepper, cilantro, broccoli flowerets, green olives, salt and pepper. Mix thoroughly. Divide mixture into 12 medium-sized, greased muffin tins and bake at 400° F for 15 minutes. Remove from oven and cool. Serve immediately or wrap and freeze for grab-and-go protein options. Two muffins equal one serving.

Terrific Tarragon Chicken Salad Pita

Ingredients

chicken breasts, boneless	2-4 oz.
celery, chopped	½ cup
fresh tarragon, chopped	1 tsp.
raisins	¼ cup
white onion, diced	2 tbsp.
low-fat mayonnaise	2 tsp.
whole-grain pitas	2
tomatoes, diced	¼ cup
romaine lettuce, chopped	¼ cup
honey mustard	2 tsp.
extra virgin olive oil	1 tbsp.

Directions

Slice chicken breasts into ½-inch cubes and pan fry in olive oil until thoroughly cooked for about 8 minutes. Refrigerate and allow to cool. In a medium-sized mixing bowl, combine cooked chicken with onions, tarragon, raisins and mayonnaise. Mix thoroughly.

Spoon chicken salad mixture into pitas. Top with tomatoes, romaine lettuce and drizzle with honey mustard. Wrap and serve. Serves 2.

Salmon Dill Wraps

This is a very quick and easy recipe that is loaded with fresh taste (the dill!), Omega-3 fats and high-quality protein.

Ingredients	
salmon	7.5-oz. can
celery, chopped	¼ cup
white onions, chopped	2 tbsp.
low-fat mayonnaise	2 tsp.
lemon or lemon, juice	¼
fresh dill, chopped	1 tsp.
salt	¼ tsp.
pepper	¼ tsp.
whole-grain wraps, small	2
tomato, diced	¼ cup
romaine lettuce, chopped	½ cup

Directions

Open can of salmon and drain juice. In a medium-sized mixing bowl, combine salmon, mayonnaise, celery, onions salt, pepper, dill and lemon juice. Mix thoroughly with a fork. Divide mixture evenly on small whole-grain wraps. Top with lettuce and tomato. Fold wraps and enjoy! Serves 2.

Chicken Breast Sandwich Supreme

This recipe is an old family favorite and can be served as a hearty lunch or satisfying dinner.

Ingredients

chicken breasts, boneless	4 oz.
whole-grain bread	4 slices
honey mustard	2 tsp.
olive oil	1 tsp.
cilantro, chopped	2 tbsp.
tarragon	1 tsp.
salt	¼ tsp.
black pepper	¼ tsp.
tomato slices	4
avocado	½

Directions

Coat chicken breasts in olive oil and sprinkle with tarragon, salt and pepper. Grill on BBQ on medium-high heat, 8 minutes on each side, or broil in oven for 6 minutes on each side.

Toast bread, add chicken and garnish with honey mustard, chopped cilantro, tomato slices and sliced avocado. Serves 2.

Veggie Pepperoni Sandwich Supreme

This sandwich is perfect for the vegetarian who still loves a great "meaty" sandwich. The secret ingredient in this sandwich is the fresh taste of cilantro.

Ingredients

Stonemill sprouted grain bread	4 slices
veggie pepperoni	6 slices
tomatoes	4 slices
seedless cucumber	8 slices
red onion, thinly sliced	2 slices
cilantro, finely chopped	2 tbsp.
low-fat mayonnaise	2 tsp.
Dijon mustard	2 tsp.

Directions

Toast bread. Coat bottom slice of each sandwich with low-fat mayonnaise and Dijon mustard. Top each sandwich with 3 slices of pepperoni, 2 slices of tomatoes, 1 slice of red onion, 4 slices of cucumber and 1 tbsp. of cilantro. Cover with second piece of whole-grain toast, cut in half diagonally. Serves 2.

Mandarin Garden Chicken Salad

If you like a salad with a bit of a sweet taste, this poppy seed dressing mixed with mandarin orange is a great combination. As a protein option, boneless, skinless chicken breast is the perfect addition to this tasty summer salad.

Ingredients

Poppy Seed Dressing

wine vinegar	1 tbsp.
Dijon mustard	½ tsp.
salt	¼ tsp.
cayenne pepper	pinch
honey	1 tbsp.
extra virgin olive	3 tbsp.
poppy seeds	1½ tsp.

Directions

Combine ingredients in mixing bowl and whisk until fully mixed. Refrigerate.

Salad

chicken breasts, boneless	2-4 oz.
poultry seasoning	1 tsp.
olive oil	2 tsp.
salt	½ tsp.
romaine lettuce, bite-sized pieces	4 cups
red onion, thinly sliced	2 tbsp.
walnuts	2 tbsp.
mandarin orange slices	6-oz. can
red pepper, thinly sliced	½
seedless cucumber, diced	¼ cup

Directions

Brush chicken breasts with olive oil, coat with salt and poultry seasoning. Broil in oven for 6 minutes on each side, or cook in BBQ on medium-high heat for 8 minutes on each side. Wrap in aluminum foil and leave in warming oven until salad is served.

In mixing bowl, combine romaine lettuce, red onion, walnuts, red pepper and cucumber. Open can of mandarin orange slices and drain, add to salad and toss. Evenly divide salad between two plates. Take chicken from warning oven, slice thinly and place on top of each salad. Drizzle with poppy seed dressing. Serves 2.

Whole-Grain Pasta and Tuna Salad

For a lower GI rating and a greater amount of fiber, whenever selecting pasta or bread, opt for whole grain. To lower the GI rating even more, cook your pasta el dente (slightly undercooked by 1 to 2 minutes).

Ingredients

light tuna	2-6 oz. cans
rotini pasta, whole grain	8-oz. package
celery, chopped	½ cup
cilantro, finely chopped	¼ cup
white onion, diced	¼ cup
olive oil	4 tbsp.
wine vinegar	2 tbsp.
lemon juice	¼ cup
salt	½ tsp.
pepper	½ tsp.
tomatoes, diced	½ cup
sugar.	1 tbsp.
cayenne pepper	¼ tsp.
red pepper	¼ cup

Directions

In a medium-sized pot, cook pasta (undercook by 2 minutes). Cool for 5 minutes in cold water. Drain and set aside. Open cans of tuna and drain. Empty tuna into large mixing bowl and break up with a fork. Add cooled pasta noodles and combine with celery, cilantro, white onion, red pepper, olive oil, wine vinegar, lemon juice, salt, pepper, diced tomatoes, sugar and cayenne pepper. Mix thoroughly, refrigerate and serve when desired. Serves 4.

Dinners

Dinner Options

Broccoliflower Pasta

Everyone loves pasta! The following recipe is aimed at satisfying the palate and the love of pasta at the same time. The combination of broccoli and cauliflower are used to replace the pasta noodles. In all pasta dishes the flavor comes from the sauce and seasoning, not from the pasta itself.

Ingredients

cauliflower	1½ cup
broccoli	1½ cup
white onion, diced	½ cup
fresh white button mushrooms, sliced	1 cup
butter	1 tsp.
tomato-based pasta sauce	1 cup
parmesan cheese	2 tsp.
garlic, fresh minced	1 tsp.
pepper	¼ tsp.
chicken or firm tofu	8 oz.

Directions

Cut broccoli and cauliflower into bite sized flowerets. Place in steamer and cook for 15 to 17 minutes until they become tender. Sautée the onions, mushrooms, fresh minced garlic and pepper with 1 tsp. of butter on medium-high heat. If adding chicken, sauté until fully cooked (approximately 8 minutes) in non-stick, lightly oiled frying pan and add to pasta sauce. If you are choosing the tofu option, cut into 1-inch cubes and add to pasta sauce before heating.

Remove broccoli and cauliflower from steamer and divide evenly between serving plates. Top with sautéed onions and mushrooms and pasta sauce with chicken or tofu, dividing evenly. Sprinkle parmesan cheese over top and enjoy! Serves 2.

Squashed Spaghetti

Spaghetti squash, appropriately named, provides a great alternative to white spaghetti noodles. Cooked properly, this vegetable has a similar consistency to spaghetti noodles along with valuable nutrition. But perhaps the best aspect of this squash is that nature provides its own dish to serve it in!

Ingredients

spaghetti squash	2 lbs.
white onion, diced	½ cup
black olives	¼ cup
tomato-based pasta sauce	1 cup
butter	1 tsp.
garlic, fresh minced	1 tsp.
pepper	¼ tsp.
oregano	1 tsp.
lean ground chicken	8 oz.
(or veggie ground meat alternative)	

Directions

Cut spaghetti squash lengthwise, scrape out seed compartment and discard. Place half of squash open side up in baking dish. Sprinkle oregano and garlic evenly over the squash, cover with aluminum foil and bake at 400° F for 1 hour and 15 minutes.

Meanwhile, in a fry pan, sautée onions and olives in butter until tender. Add protein option of lean ground chicken or veggie meat alternative to fry pan and stir until fully cooked. Heat tomato-based pasta sauce and add to mixture of sautéed onions, black olives and protein option.

When the squash is done, remove aluminum foil and with a large fork, scoop out the squash from shell. The flesh of the squash should be stringy but tender, similar to spaghetti. As an interesting twist, rather than placing the squash on a plate, return it to the shell for serving. Divide sauce mix evenly over the squash. Serves 2.

Tofu Vegetable Medley Salad

Served cold, this salad is a summertime favorite. Vegetables should only be lightly steamed so they retain their crunch.

Ingredients

broccoli flowerets	1 cup
sliced carrots	½ cup
cauliflower flowerets	1 cup
white onions, diced	¼ cup
mushrooms, sliced	½ cup
raisins	½ cup
red peppers, diced	¼ cup
black olives, sliced	¼ cup
balsamic vinegar	¼ cup
sugar	1 tbsp.
fresh cilantro, finely chopped	¼ cup
olive oil	¼ cup
tofu, cut into small cubes	500 g

Directions

Place cut-up broccoli, carrots and cauliflower in a steamer and steam for 15 minutes; then rinse in cold water until chilled. Drain and combine with onions, mushrooms, raisins, red pepper, black olives, balsamic vinegar, sugar, cilantro, olive oil and tofu. Mix thoroughly. Place in refrigerator and chill. Serves 4.

Warm Chili Salad

This recipe is great for vegetarians or meat-lovers, depending on your preference. You can freeze this chili in small Tupperware containers for quick and easy lunch options at work. Perfect on a cold winter's day!

Ingredients

crushed tomatoes	19-oz. can
kidney beans	14-oz. can
black beans	14-oz. can
pinto beans	14-oz. can
tomato paste	3-oz. can
veggie ground meat alternative or ground chicken	½ pound
celery, diced	¼ cup
white onions, diced	4 tbsp.
chili powder	3 tbsp.
garlic powder	1 tsp.
cumin	1 tsp.
salt	½ tsp.
pepper	½ tsp.
sugar	2 tsp.
romaine lettuce, rough cut	8 cups
whole-grain or baked nacho chips, broken	1 cup

Directions

Combine crushed tomatoes, kidney beans, black beans, pinto beans (rinsed), tomato paste, veggie meat alternative (ground soy) or cooked ground chicken, celery, onions, chili powder, cumin, garlic powder, salt, pepper and sugar in a large pot. Bring to a boil, reduce to simmer and cook for 45 minutes.

Wash and place romaine lettuce on plates. Spoon 1 cup of chili mixture over the salad, top with remaining broken nacho chips and enjoy. Serves 6.

Perfect Portobello Burger

We all love a good hamburger. Unfortunately, eating too much red meat can result in inflammatory diseases such as arthritis , unnecessary weight gain and compromised digestion. One of the great vegetarian kitchen secrets is replacing a regular meat patty with a Portobello mushroom which provides much of the flavor and consistency of a beef hamburger.

Ingredients

portobello mushrooms, stems removed	2 large
whole-grain buns	2
low-fat Swiss cheese	2 slices
garlic powder	½ tsp.
butter	2 tsp.
hot sauce	2 tsp.
tomato slices	4
romaine lettuce, chopped	½ cup
red onions	2 slices
Dijon mustard	2 tsp.
green relish	2 tsp.

Directions

Preheat oven to 400° F. Rinse mushrooms caps first and pat dry with a paper towel. Place mushroom caps, gill side up on non-stick baking sheet. Top with butter, hot sauce and garlic powder. Broil for 6 minutes. Remove and top mushrooms with cheese slices and return to oven for 1 to 2 minutes until cheese is melted. Slice whole-grain buns in half and toast. Place cooked mushroom caps on bottom of bun and garnish with Dijon mustard, green relish, sliced red onions, tomato slices and lettuce. Add top bun and enjoy! Serves 2.

Pesto Tilapia with Fresh Tomato Salad

Tilapia is among the easiest and tastiest fish you can prepare. Combined with the fresh tomato-pesto salad, this meal will leave you feeling satisfied and provide the perfect nutritional combination of protein, fat and carbohydrates.

Ingredients

tilapia fillets	2-6 oz.
tomato, diced	1 cup
cucumber, diced	1 cup
white onion, diced	¼ cup
salt	¼ tsp.
pepper	¼ tsp.
parsley, finely chopped	¼ tsp.
red pepper, diced	¼ cup

Low-Fat Basil Pesto

fresh basil	1½ cups
garlic	4 cloves
pine nuts	¼ cup
parmesan cheese, grated	¼ cup
lemon juice	⅛ cup
extra virgin olive oil	⅛ cup

Directions

Pesto

Mix basil, garlic, pine nuts and Parmesan cheese together in the food processor. Once all ingredients are blended well, drizzle in lemon and oil, mixing until blended. Set aside.

Fish

Place tilapia filets in greased baking dish. Sprinkle with salt and pepper. Spoon 1 tsp. pesto over top of each fillet and bake at 400° F for 25 minutes. In a mixing bowl combine tomato, cucumber, white onion, parsley and red pepper. Spoon remaining pesto sauce over top and lightly toss. Place in refrigerator. When ready to serve, place tilapia fillets on plates and spoon tomato salad on the side. Serves 2.

Blackened Red Snapper with Steamed Spinach

If spice is what you crave, this dish is definitely for you. Blackening spice is a great way to ramp up any meal and is perfect with red snapper. This meal doesn't take long to prepare and will take you from the ordinary to the extraordinary. The more coating you leave on each fillet, the hotter the taste. Bon appetite!

Ingredients

snapper fillets, skinless	2-5 oz.
Crimini mushrooms, sliced	½ cup
orange, cut into wedges	1 medium
spinach, fresh	1 medium package
white onions, diced	½ cup
butter	2 tsp.
garlic powder	1 tsp.
salt	½ tsp.

Blackening Spices

paprika	½ tbsp.
thyme	¼ tsp.
oregano	¼ tsp.
onion powder or onion salt (if onion salt, use a little less)	1 tsp.
salt	1½ tsp.
cayenne pepper	½ tsp.
white pepper	½ tsp.
black pepper	½ tsp.

Directions

Combine blackening spices in a flat mixing bowl and mix thoroughly; set aside.

Sautée mushroom and onions with garlic powder in 1 tsp. butter for 5 minutes. Wash and steam spinach in steamer until wilted (approximately 2 minutes). Do not overcook. Melt remaining butter and dip snapper fillets until fully coated. Heat a large cast iron skillet to high heat, dip coated fillets in blackening spices and cook for 2 minutes on each side. Keeping the fillets in the pan pour 3 tbsp. of water in pan and cover for 1 minute. Place steamed spinach on plates and top with sautéed mushrooms and onions. Place blackened fillets on top, garnish with orange wedges and enjoy! Serves 2.

Peach-Mango BBQ Chicken

This delicious BBQ meal will make your guests think they were ordering from the best restaurant in town! Easy to make, naturally sweet and high in protein—bon appetite!

Ingredients

chicken breasts, boneless/skinless	3-4 oz.
poultry seasoning	2 tsp.
sweet potatoes, small	4
butter	2 tsp.
mango, diced	2
fresh peaches, diced	2
white onion, diced	½ cup
fresh cilantro, finely chopped	½ cup
sugar	1 tbsp.
jalapeno pepper, finely chopped	1 tbsp.
salt	½ tsp.
pepper	½ tsp.
tomato	8 slices
seedless cucumber	16 slices
olive oil	4 tsp.

Directions

Peel mango and peaches, remove pits, dice and place in a mixing bowl. Add cilantro, white onion, sugar and jalapeno into bowl and stir until fully mixed. Place ¼ of the mixture in a small mixing bowl and rough chop with an electronic hand blender or in food processor. Do not purée. Set aside. Peel and cut sweet potatoes into 2-inch cubes and place in steamer for 30 minutes. Remove, add butter and mash. Place in warming oven at 250° F. Coat chicken breast with olive oil, salt, pepper and poultry seasoning. Cook (broil in the oven for 6 mins on each side) or BBQ on medium-high heat for 8 minutes on each side. Spoon on 1 tbsp. of blended chutney mixture and continue to cook on low heat for 5 minutes. Divide mashed sweet potato evenly in the center of each plate. Place chicken breast on top and cover with balance of chutney. Garnish with tomato and cucumber slices and enoy! Serves 4.

Stuffed Chicken Breasts over Asparagus Spears

Ingredients

chicken breast, boneless skinless	2-5 oz.
apples, sliced	½ cup
walnuts, crushed	2 tbsp.
low-fat Swiss cheese	2 slices
butter	1 tsp.
asparagus spears	1 lb.
poultry seasoning	2 tsp.
salt	½ tsp.
pepper	½ tsp.

Directions

With a sharp knife, butterfly each chicken breast in half. Open flat and place between waxed paper and pound flat with a meat mallet. Remove from waxed paper. Coat chicken with 2 tsp. of melted butter; then sprinkle with 2 tsp. of poultry seasoning, salt and pepper on all sides. On ½ of each chicken breast place ½ of the sliced apples, crushed walnuts and Swiss cheese slice. Fold over top half of chicken breasts. Secure sides with tooth picks. Place in baking dish and bake at 400° F for 45 minutes. When fully cooked, prick the chicken breasts with a fork: the liquid coming from chicken breasts should be clear.

While the chicken breasts are baking, wash asparagus and break off approximately 1 inch from the bottom of each spear. About 10 minutes prior to the chicken breasts being done, place asparagus in steamer and cook for 10 minutes. Be careful not to overcook asparagus as it can become soft very quickly. Divide asparagus spears evenly on two plates. Add salt and pepper. Place cooked stuffed chicken breasts on top of asparagus. Enjoy! Serves 2.

Curried Chicken with Vegetables

Flavor, flavor and more flavor. One of the great combinations in culinary history is curry and pineapple. This "meal in a pan" will fill your kitchen and your home with the delicious fragrance of curry and will no doubt become a favorite with your family and friends.

Ingredients

chicken thighs and drumsticks	1 ½ pounds
white onions, sliced	¼ cup
Crimini mushrooms, sliced	¼ cup
bok choy, chopped	½ cup
broccoli flowerets	½ cup
carrots, sliced	½ cup
curry powder	1 tsp.
curry paste	½ tsp.
brown sugar	1 tbsp.
coconut milk	8 oz.
chicken stock	4 oz.
corn starch	1 tbsp.
fresh pineapple, chopped	½ cup

Directions

In a saucepan cook curry powder and curry paste over medium-low heat for about 2 minutes. Pour the coconut milk into the pan and mix well. Stir in brown sugar and chicken stock. Add the onions, broccoli, chicken, mushrooms and bok choy. Bring the mixture to a boil; then reduce to low heat and simmer for 25 minutes. Meanwhile, whisk 1 tbsp. of corn starch with 2 to 3 tbsp. of water. Stir mixture into the pot. Mix in pineapple and continue cooking until the mixture thickens. Serve and enjoy! Serves 4.

Mama's Homemade Burgers

The key to creating a healthier burger is to use extra-lean ground beef. The difference in fat content is quite substantial. Regular ground beef tips the scale at 30 percent fat content, while extra-lean ground beef's fat content is 10 percent or less. If you drain the fat after cooking extra-lean beef, the fat content drops to approximately 5 percent.

Ingredients

extra-lean ground beef	6 oz.
whole-grain bread crumbs	½ cup
garlic powder	¼ cup
white onion, finely chopped	2 tbsp.
salt	½ tsp.
pepper	½ tsp.
worcestershire sauce	2 tsp.
omega-3 egg	1

Directions

In a mixing bowl combine extra-lean ground beef, bread crumbs, egg, diced onion, salt, pepper, Worcestershire sauce and garlic powder. Mix thoroughly and kneed until consistency allows you to make it into a patty. Divide mixture into 2 patties. Place on high heat on BBQ for 2 minutes on each side to sear the burgers. Reduce heat to medium and cook for 5 minutes on each side. Enjoy with a side salad. Serves 2.

Herbalicious!

As mentioned, we are big fans of eating fresh herbs in our family. The tasty herbs and spices described below can infuse your food with bursting flavor. While fresh is always best, if all else fails, dried spices are a good second choice. My top five herbs are:

- Coriander/Cilantro
- Basil
- Dill
- Oregano
- Garlic

Coriander/Cilantro

Coriander is a green leafy herb that is also known as cilantro. When looking for coriander in your local grocery store, the leaf bears a strong resemblance to Italian flat leaf parsley. Fresh coriander is highly perishable and should be kept in the fridge wrapped in a damp cloth or paper towel. It should last between 3 to 5 days. If not buying fresh leaves, purchase whole coriander seeds instead of coriander powder. Coriander powder tends to lose its flavor quickly. Coriander seeds can easily be ground with a mortar and pestle.

Studies have shown coriander to be beneficial in blood sugar control, to have anti-bacterial effects and to be rich in phytonutrients (plant chemicals that offer disease-preventing properties). This fresh and tasty herb also offers a very good source of dietary fiber and a good source of iron and magnesium.

Basil

From pizza to tomato sauces, basil can enhance the taste of many dishes. Basil has gained enormous popularity as the main ingredient of pesto. Similar to dill, basil can be eaten fresh or chopped up and frozen for future use. In addition to basil's delicious taste, it has also been shown to have anti-bacterial and anti-inflammatory properties. An added bonus is that it is chock full of nutrition containing vitamin K, calcium, iron, vitamin A and fiber. There are several different types of basil; try including lemon basil, red basil, anise or cinnamon basil in your diet.

Dill

Dill is one of my family's favorite spices and is the perfect match for fish (salmon), in salad dressings, e.g., cucumber dill dressing, or in soups. Fresh dill has a soft, sweet taste. When looking for dill in the grocery store, its leaves appear quite wispy and fernlike and may appear slightly wilted, as they usually drop right after being picked. Fresh dill will keep in your refrigerator for 2 to 3 days. It can also be chopped and frozen in air-tight containers or in small ice cube trays for use in soups or stews. Dried dill seeds are also available and can be used instead of fresh dill. Dill offers a very good source of iron and is a good source of calcium and manganese.

Oregano

Oregano is a light green herb that is a member of the mint family. This ever-popular herb is a flavor enhancer to pizza, omelets, vegetables and fish. Recently, you may have seen "oil of oregano" in your local health food store. The oils derived from oregano have been shown to demonstrate impressive and potent anti-oxidant and anti-bacterial properties. Oregano also contains fiber, iron, manganese, calcium and vitamin C.

Garlic

Garlic is one of the oldest known medicinal plants. This humble clove is used around the world as a delicious flavoring agent for many dishes, including garlic bread, pasta sauces, poultry and stir-fries. The health benefits of garlic have also been well touted for centuries. For example, raw garlic has been used as a natural antibiotic, effective against some strains of harmful bacteria. Garlic is also useful for decreasing blood pressure and cholesterol, removing heavy metals from the body, preventing cancer and acting as an antifungal and antiviral agent. One clove of garlic contains vitamins A, B and C, selenium, iodine, potassium, iron, calcium, zinc and magnesium.

Sweetening It Up with Spices!

There are many ways to add sweet-tasting spices to your food without adding calories or causing blood sugar fluctuations. The top five sweet-tasting spices are:

Ginger

For thousands of years, ginger has been used to treat a number of ailments such as bloating, coughing, vomiting, diarrhea and rheumatism. The active ingredient in ginger is gingerol, a compound that's thought to relax blood vessels, stimulate blood flow and relieve pain. Ginger can be used freshly ground in a number of seafood, meat or vegetable dishes. It is also a wonderful addition to deserts and baking (i.e. ginger bread cookies or on top of yogurt). For stomach upset, ginger tea is very soothing.

Cinnamon

Research has shown cinnamon to have numerous health benefits including being anti-inflammatory, helping to balance blood sugar naturally for type II diabetes and having anti-bacterial and anti-fungal properties. In addition, cinnamon is a wonderful addition to dishes and desserts and can help to satisfy any sweet tooth. Cinnamon is available in ground form or in sticks. The fragrant and sweet taste of cinnamon is the perfect taste over the winter months!

Nutmeg

Nutmeg has a sweet, spicy and nutty taste which makes it a favorite for desserts such as pumpkin pies, puddings and cookies. In addition, nutmeg can be added to apple cider, stewed fruits, chutney, meats, soups, sauces and vegetables.

From a health perspective, nutmeg has also been shown to be beneficial for relieving nausea and appears to aid in digestion.

Vanilla

Vanilla is one of the most widely used flavors in the world. Vanilla is used in many desert recipes for its smooth and soothing taste. It is available as vanilla beans or as vanilla extract. In addition, many tea companies now offer delicious vanilla chai teas that are perfect for curbing cravings.

Dark Chocolate Shavings

For all chocolate lovers out there—it is wonderful news that dark chocolate is good for overall health. Filled to the brim with anti-oxidants, dark chocolate shavings over warm drinks, fruits, yogurts or puddings are just what the doctor ordered!

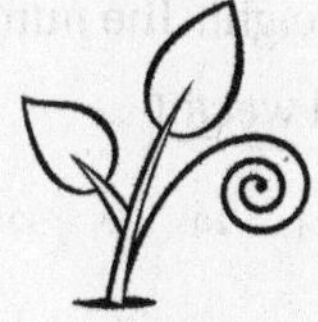

Appendix

"We are indeed much more than what we eat, but what we eat can nevertheless help us to be much more than what we are."

Adele Davis, (1904-1974)
American pioneer in the field of nutrition

Chapter 1

Body Mass Index

To use the table, find the appropriate height in the left-hand column. Move across the row to the given weight. The number at the top of the column is the BMI for that height and weight

BMI (kg/m2)	19	20	21	22	23	24	25	26	27	28	29	30	35	40
Height (in.)	Weight (lb.)													
58	91	96	100	105	110	115	119	124	129	134	138	143	167	191
59	94	99	104	109	114	119	124	128	133	138	143	148	173	198
60	97	102	107	112	118	123	128	133	138	143	148	153	179	204
61	100	106	111	116	122	127	132	137	143	148	153	158	185	211
62	104	109	115	120	126	131	136	142	147	153	158	164	191	218
63	107	113	118	124	130	135	141	146	152	158	163	169	197	225
64	110	116	122	128	134	140	145	151	157	163	169	174	204	232
65	114	120	126	132	138	144	150	156	162	168	174	180	210	240
66	118	124	130	136	142	148	155	161	167	173	179	186	216	247
67	121	127	134	140	146	153	159	166	172	178	185	191	223	255
68	125	131	138	144	151	158	164	171	177	184	190	197	230	262
69	128	135	142	149	155	162	169	176	182	189	196	203	236	270
70	132	139	146	153	160	167	174	181	188	195	202	207	243	278
71	136	143	150	157	165	172	179	186	193	200	208	215	250	286
72	140	147	154	162	169	177	184	191	199	206	213	221	258	294
73	144	151	159	166	174	182	189	197	204	212	219	227	265	302
74	148	155	163	171	179	186	194	202	210	218	225	233	272	311
75	152	160	168	176	184	192	200	208	216	224	232	240	279	319
76	156	164	172	180	189	197	205	213	221	230	238	246	287	328

BMI Categories

- Underweight = <18.5
- Normal weight = 18.5–24.9
- Overweight = 25–29.9
- Obesity = BMI of 30 or greater

Risk of Associated Disease According to BMI and Waist Size

BMI		Waist less than or equal to 40 in. (men) or 35 in. (women)	Waist greater than 40 in. (men) or 35 in. (women)
18.5 or less	Underweight	-	-
18.5–24.9	Normal		-
25.0–29.9	Overweight	Increased	High
30.0–34.9	Obese	High	Very High
35.0–39.9	Obese	Very High	Very High
40 or greater	Extremely Obese	Extremely High	Extremely High

Chapter 2

Waist-to-Hip Ratio Chart

Your health is not only affected by how much body fat you have, but also by where most of the fat is located on your body. People who tend to gain weight mostly in their hips and buttocks have a pear body shape, while people who tend to gain weight mostly in the abdomen have more of an apple body shape.

If you have an apple-shaped body, you are at increased risk for the health problems associated with obesity, such as Type 2 diabetes, coronary heart disease and high blood pressure. Fortunately, with proper dietary control and exercise management, your risk can be reduced dramatically.

It's very simple to calculate your waist-to-hip ratio, using a soft measuring tape such as those used for sewing, and a calculator.

1. Measure your waist circumference at the narrowest part. Do not pull the tape too tight.
2. Measure your hip circumference at its widest part.
3. On your calculator, divide waist measurement by hip measurement.
4. For example, if your waist is 35" and your hips are 41", then divide 35 by 41, and your calculator will give you a reading of 0.85. This is the waist-to-hip ratio (or WHR).

Waist to Hip Ratios

Male	Female	Health Risk Based Solely on WHR
0.95 or below	0.80 or below	Low Risk
0.96 to 1.0	0.81 to 0.85	Moderate Risk
1.0+	0.85+	High Risk

Height and Weight Tables of the Metropolitan Life Insurance Company for Women

Height in Shoes	Small Frame	Medium Frame	Large Frame
6'	138 to 151 lb.	148 to 162 lb.	158 to 179 lb.
5'11"	135 to 148 lb.	145 to 159 lb.	155 to 176 lb.
5'10"	132 to 145 lb.	142 to 156 lb.	152 to 173 lb.
5'9"	129 to 142 lb.	139 to 153 lb.	149 to 170 lb.
5'8"	126 to 139 lb.	136 to 150 lb.	146 to 167 lb.
5'7"	123 to 136 lb.	133 to 147 lb.	143 to 163 lb.
5'6"	120 to 133 lb.	130 to 144 lb.	140 to 159 lb.
5'5"	117 to 130 lb.	127 to 141 lb.	137 to 155 lb.
5'4"	114 to 127 lb.	124 to 138 lb.	134 to 151 lb.
5'3"	111 to 124 lb.	121 to 135 lb.	131 to 147 lb.
5'2"	108 to 121 lb.	118 to 132 lb.	128 to 143 lb.
5'1"	106 to 118 lb.	115 to 129 lb.	125 to 140 lb.
5'	104 to 115 lb.	113 to 126 lb.	122 to 137 lb.
4'11"	103 to 113 lb.	111 to 123 lb.	120 to 134 lb.
4'10"	102 to 111 lb.	109 to 121 lb.	118 to 131 lb.

Please note: The ideal weights given in these tables are for ages 25 to 59. The weights assume you are wearing shoes with 1-inch heels and indoor clothing weighing 3 pounds.

Height and Weight Tables of the Metropolitan Life Insurance Company for Men

Height in Shoes	Small Frame	Medium Frame	Large Frame
6'4"	162 to 176 lb.	171 to 187 lb.	181 to 207 lb.
6'3"	158 to 172 lb.	167 to 182 lb.	176 to 202 lb.
6'2"	155 to 168 lb.	164 to 178 lb.	172 to 197 lb.
6'1"	152 to 164 lb.	160 to 174 lb.	168 to 192 lb.
6'	149 to 160 lb.	157 to 170 lb.	164 to 188 lb.
5'11"	146 to 157 lb.	154 to 166 lb.	161 to 184 lb.
5'10"	144 to 154 lb.	151 to 163 lb.	158 to 180 lb.
5'9"	142 to 151 lb.	148 to 160 lb.	155 to 176 lb.
5'8"	140 to 148 lb.	145 to 157 lb.	152 to 172 lb.
5'7"	138 to 145 lb.	142 to 154 lb.	149 to 168 lb.
5'6"	136 to 142 lb.	139 to 151 lb.	146 to 164 lb.
5'5"	134 to 140 lb.	137 to 148 lb.	144 to 160 lb.
5'4"	132 to 138 lb.	135 to 145 lb.	142 to 156 lb.
5'3"	130 to 136 lb.	133 to 143 lb.	140 to 153 lb.
5'2"	128 to 134 lb.	131 to 141 lb.	138 to 150 lb.

How to Measure Percentage of Body Fat Using the U.S. Navy Method

- Measure your height, without shoes, in inches or centimeters
- Measure the circumference around your abdomen at the horizontal level of the navel.
- Measure the circumference of the neck, below the larynx, with the tape sloping slightly downward to the front.
- For women only: measure the circumference of the hips at the largest horizontal measure.

For Men

Measurement in Centimeters:

% Fat = 495/(1.0324 – .19077(LOG(abdomen-neck)) + .15456(LOG(height))) – 450

Or

Measurement in Inches:

% Fat = (86.010*LOG((abdomen) – (neck))) – (70.041*LOG(height)) + 36.76

For Women

Measurement in Centimeters:

% Fat = 495/(1.29579 – .35004(LOG(abdomen+hip – neck)) + .22100(LOG(height))) – 450

Measurement in Inches:

% Fat = (163.205*LOG((abdomen) + (hip) – (neck))) – (97.684*LOG(height)) –78.387

Chapter 6

Gluten-Free/Wheat-Free Grains

Gluten is a protein found in grains such as wheat, barely, rye, spelt and kamut. In the United States alone, over 3 million people suffer from celiac disease. Celiac disease is an autoimmune form of gluten intolerance that can trigger a myriad of symptoms such as abdominal cramping, diarrhea, weight loss, energy loss, irritability, depression, joint pain and a host of other additional complaints If diagnosed with celiac disease, a strict gluten-free diet must be maintained for life.

Other people may experience a sensitivity or allergy to wheat. If this is the case, a wheat-free diet should also be followed. That said, certain individuals who are sensitive to wheat (not gluten) can still include distinct relatives of wheat such as spelt or kamut in their diet.

Grains with gluten include:

- Wheat (including varieties such as spelt, kamut, durum, semolina, bulgur)
- Barely
- Rye
- Triticale (a wheat hybrid)
- Oats

The following are some foods that may contain gluten:

- Bran
- Cola drinks
- Graham flour
- Malt
- Millet
- Prepared mustard
- Oats
- Root beer
- Rye seeds or flour
- Salad dressings (many prepared types; read the ingredient panel)
- Soups and sauces that use flour as a thickener
- Soy sauce
- Wheat and wheat products
- Worcestershire sauce
- Distilled white vinegar

Grains without gluten include:

- Amaranth
- Buckwheat
- Corn
- Millet
- Quinoa
- Rice
- Teff
- Wild rice

Oats are generally gluten-free but can be contaminated with wheat during the growing or processing of the grain. If following a gluten-free diet, check with your doctor first.

Chapter 10

Food Additives, Colorings and Preservatives to Avoid

Acesulfame-K	Commercially sold as Sunette or Sweet One and found in numerous diet products and beverages. This artificial sweetener is 180–200 times sweeter than sugar. Although approved by the FDA in 1988, studies have indicated that Acesulfame K causes cancer in lab animals.
Artificial colors	In the United States, FD&C (food, drug and cosmetic) colors are given numbers to approve the synthetic food dye that does not exist in nature. The colors approved are: Blue No. 1 Brilliant Blue FCF, E133 (Blue shade) Blue No. 2 Indigotine, E132 (Dark Blue shade) Green No. 3 Fast Green FCF, E143 (Bluish green shade) Red No. 40 Allura Red AC, E129 (Red shade) Red No. 3 Erythrosine, E127 (Pink shade) Yellow No. 5 Tartrazine, E102 (Yellow shade) Yellow No. 6 Sunset Yellow FCF, E110 (Orange shade Most of the colors are derived from coal tar and must be certified by the FDA not to contain more than 10 ppm of lead and arsenic. Tartrazine has been shown to be indicated in hives, asthma and behavioral issues. Erthrosine has been linked to thyroid tumors in rats. Other artificial colors are suspected to cause associated symptoms such as hyperactivity and depression and may be carcinogenic (cancer causing).
Aspartame	Aspartame is an artificial sweetener found in over 6,000 food and beverages worldwide and is also marketed as Equal or Nutrasweet. Studies have indicated possible connections with aspartame and brain tumors, headaches, brain lesions and lymphoma.
BHT & BHA	Butylated hydroxyanisole (BHA) and the related compound butylated hydroxytoluene (BHT) are phenolic compounds that are often added to foods to preserve fats. Animal studies have shown the potential link between BHA/BHT and cancer.
Monosodium glutamate	A flavor enhancer found in soups, salad dressings, chips, frozen entrees and restaurant foods. Studies have shown some people to be extremely sensitive to MSG and have linked it to headaches, nausea, weakness, burning sensations in the back of neck and forearms, wheezing, changes in heart rate and difficulty breathing. After earlier studies demonstrated MSG destroyed nerve cells in the brains of mice, it was banned from baby food.
Sodium nitrates (or nitrites)	Sodium nitrite is used as a preservative and to preserve color in pink meats such as bacon, ham, hot dogs, luncheon meats, corn beef and smoked fish. These additives can lead to the formation of cancer causing chemicals called nitrosamines.

Recommended Daily Allowance (RDA) vs. Optimal Daily Allowance (ODA)

	RDA	ODA
Vitamin A	1,000 mcg	7, 000–10,000 mcg (I.U.)
Vitamin D	200 I.U.	1000 I.U.
Vitamin E	15 I.U.	400 I.U.
Vitamin K	80 mcg	60–80 mcg
Vitamin B 1 (thiamine)	1.5mg	50–100 mg
Vitamin B 2 (riboflavin)	1.7 mg	50 mg
Vitamin B 3 (niacin)	19 mg	50mg
Vitamin B 5 (panthothenic acid)	7 mg	200–400 mg
Vitamin B6	2 mg	50mg–200 mg
Folic acid	200 mcg	400–800 mcg
Vitamin C	60 mg	1,000-7,000 mg
Calcium	800 mg	500mg–1,200 mg
Chloride	750 mg	Not usually recommended
Chromium	50–200 mcg	200–400 mcg
Magnesium	350 mg	500–100 mg
Potassium	2,000 mg	100 mg
Selenium	70 mcg	200 mcg
Zinc	15 mg	25 mg

Source: http://www.hsph.harvard.edu/nutritionsource/vitamins.html

The Last 15 Food Journal: Day 1

Please note: You may photocopy this food journal and use for as many days as you like. You need to keep a food journal for a minimum of three consecutive days to get an idea what your diet is like.

Date: ____/______/____

Breakfast

Time: __________

____

____

____

Beverage: ______________________________

Lunch

Time: __________

____

____

____

Beverage: ______________________________

Dinner

Time: __________

____

____

____

Beverage: ______________________________

Snacks

Time: ______ ______________________________________

Time: ______ ______________________________________

Did you feel fatigue or sluggishness at times throughout the day? If so, when?

____

____

____

Did you eat at times when you were not hungry or for emotional reasons? If so, please describe.

____

____

____

Did you experience cravings during the day? If so, please describe at what time and how you dealt with the craving.

____

____

____

The Last 15 Food Journal: Day 2

Date: ____/______/____

Breakfast

Time: __________

____

____

____

Beverage: ____________________________________

Lunch

Time: __________

____

____

____

Beverage: ____________________________________

Dinner

Time: __________

____

____

____

Beverage: ____________________________________

Snacks

Time: ______ ____

Time: ______ ____

Did you feel fatigue or sluggishness at times throughout the day? If so, when?

____

____

____

Did you eat at times when you were not hungry or for emotional reasons? If so, please describe.

____

____

____

Did you experience cravings during the day? If so, please describe at what time and how you dealt with the craving.

____

____

____

The Last 15 Food Journal: Day 3

Date: ____/______/____

Breakfast

Time: ________

____

____

____

Beverage: _____________________________

Lunch

Time: ________

____

____

____

Beverage: _____________________________

Dinner

Time: ________

____

____

____

Beverage: _____________________________

Snacks

Time: ______ ______________________________

Time: ______ ______________________________

Did you feel fatigue or sluggishness at times throughout the day? If so, when?

____

____

____

Did you eat at times when you were not hungry or for emotional reasons? If so, please describe.

____

____

____

Did you experience cravings during the day? If so, please describe at what time and how you dealt with the craving.

____

____

____

The Last 15 Food Journal: Day 4

Date: ____/______/____

Breakfast

Time: __________

____

____

____

Beverage: ______________________________

Lunch

Time: __________

____

____

____

Beverage: ______________________________

Dinner

Time: __________

____

____

____

Beverage: ______________________________

Snacks

Time: ______ ______________________________________

Time: ______ ______________________________________

Did you feel fatigue or sluggishness at times throughout the day? If so, when?

____

____

____

Did you eat at times when you were not hungry or for emotional reasons? If so, please describe.

____

Did you experience cravings during the day? If so, please describe at what time and how you dealt with the craving.

The Last 15 Food Journal: Day 5

Date: ____/______/____

Breakfast

Time: __________

____

____

____

Beverage: ________________________________

Lunch

Time: __________

____

____

____

Beverage: ________________________________

Dinner

Time: __________

____

____

____

Beverage: ________________________________

Snacks

Time: ______ ______________________________________

Time: ______ ______________________________________

Did you feel fatigue or sluggishness at times throughout the day? If so, when?

____

____

____

Did you eat at times when you were not hungry or for emotional reasons? If so, please describe.

____

Did you experience cravings during the day? If so, please describe at what time and how you dealt with the craving.

The Last 15 Food Journal: Day 6

Date: ____/______/____

Breakfast

Time: _________

____

____

____

Beverage: ______________________________

Lunch

Time: _________

____

____

____

Beverage: ______________________________

Dinner

Time: _________

____

____

____

Beverage: ______________________________

Snacks

Time: ______ ______________________________________

Time: ______ ______________________________________

Did you feel fatigue or sluggishness at times throughout the day? If so, when?

____

____

____

Did you eat at times when you were not hungry or for emotional reasons? If so, please describe.

____

Did you experience cravings during the day? If so, please describe at what time and how you dealt with the craving.

The Last 15 Food Journal: Day 7

Date: ____/______/____

Breakfast

Time: __________

____

____

____

Beverage: ________________________________

Lunch

Time: __________

____

____

____

Beverage: ________________________________

Dinner

Time: __________

____

____

____

Beverage: ________________________________

Snacks

Time: ______ ____

Time: ______ ____

Did you feel fatigue or sluggishness at times throughout the day? If so, when?

____

____

____

Did you eat at times when you were not hungry or for emotional reasons? If so, please describe.

____

Did you experience cravings during the day? If so, please describe at what time and how you dealt with the craving.

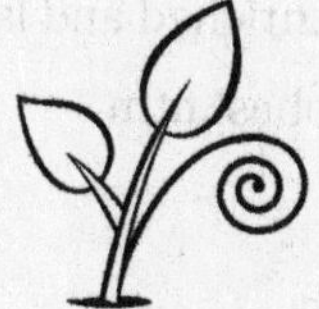

Product Resource Guide

Grocery items

Yogurt

Astro biobest yogurt contains acidophilus and bifidum cultures. Varieties include omega-3, calcium-enriched and lactose reduced.
www.astro.ca/products/biobest.htm

Tea

1. Yogi Tea: This is my favorite brand of tea. There are a variety of high quality teas to match your mood, physical wants and taste. The green teas are one of the best on the market. For more information, visit www.yogitea.com
2. Stash Premium Tea: contains a variety of high quality teas such as chai white and green tea. For more information, visit www.stashtea.com

Breads and baked goods

Stonemill Bakehouse: bread offers a variety of high quality, whole grain and low glycemic index breads including omega-3, sprouted grain and 100% spelt bread. They glycemic index of the sprouted grain bread is 55 and makes it an excellent option for The Last 15.
www.stonemillbakehouse.com
The Stonemill Bakehouse Ltd.,
426 Nugget Ave.
Toronto ON Canada
M1S 4A4
Tel: 416-757-0582 Toll Free: 877-517-8198

Fish products

Raincoast trading offers low mercury tuna, wild salmon (both canned and in smoked form). They can be reached at www.raincoasttrading.com.

Veggie burgers

Dr. Praeger's offers a delicious line of veggie burgers in Bombay, Tex Mex or California style. For more information visit www.drpraegers.com.

Soup

Imagine soup offers a variety of gourmet organic, MSG free soups and soup broths that are ready made. For more information, please visit www.imaginefoods.com.

Pure pressed juice

Black River offers a variety of high quality cold pressed juice. I recommend adding the juices to water for a sweet natural flavor. The cranberry juice is terrific for urinary tract health and is delicious! For more information, please visit www.blackriverjuice.com.

Cleaning products

Nature clean offers a line of chemical free household, laundry and cleaning products for your home. With a recent 5 year study by the Environmental Protection Agency finding concentrations of 20 toxic compounds to be as much as 200 times higher inside the homes vs. outdoors—these products are a must! For more information, please visit www.naturecleanliving.com.

Health food chains

Whole Foods Market, Inc.
www.wholefoodsmarket.com

Wild Oats Market, Inc.
www.wildoats.com

Healthy restaurant chains

Lettuce Eatery
www.lettuceeatery.com

Supplements

Genuine Health

317 Adelaide St. West, Suite 501

Toronto, Ontario M5V 1P9

Tel: (416) 977-4339 Toll Free: (877) 500-7888

Recommended products include

- *greens+ multi+*. Combines the nutrition of a green powder and a complete multi-vitamin in one.
- *multi + daily trim*—multi-vitamin specific to weight loss
- *Fish oil*—omega-3 + fit (capsules)—is made from wild fish sources. Provides distilled omega-3 fish oil in addition to metabolic boosting effects.
- *Protein powder*—proteins+ contains the highest quality alpha whey isolate protein powder. Available in chocolate or vanilla flavors.
- *abs+*—Helps to reduce waistline naturally (natural ingredients such as green tea extract and CLA) and is clinically proven to speed weight loss.

Probiotics

Bio- K+

Parc Scientifique 495 boul. Armand-Frappier

Laval (Quebec) H7V 4B3 Canada

1-800-593-BIOK

www.biokplus.com

Jarrow Formulas

Jarro dophilus EPS

www.jarrow.com

Recommended Reading

- *Eating Well for Optimum Health* by Dr. Andrew Weil
- *Eating Alive*: *Prevention Thru Good Digestion* by Dr. John Matsen
- *The Yeast Connection*: A Medical Breakthrough by William G Crook

- *The Brain Diet: The Connection Between Nutrition, Mental Health and Intelligence* by Dr. Alan Logan
- ***Foods that Heal*** by Bernard Jensen
- *How the World's Longest-Lived People Achieve Everlasting Health and How You Can Too* by Bradley J. Willcox, D. Craig Willcox , Makoto Suzuki
- *The Bone-Building Solution* by Sam Graci, Dr. Carolyn DeMarco and Dr. Leticia Rao

Other

Dr. Joey's headshots: Photography by Helen Tansey at www.helentansey.com

Dr. Joey's makeup done by: Pippa Leavy at pleavy@rogers.com

Illustrations throughout book done by: Samantha Walsh, samantha.walsh@hotmail.com

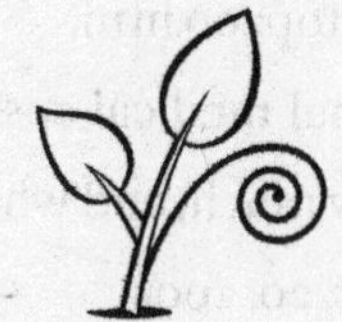

References

Chapter 1

1. G. Danaei, S et al. "Causes of cancer in the world: comparative risk assessment of nine behavioral and environmental risk factors." *The Lancet.* November 19, 2005; 366: 1784-1793.
2. http://www.rxlist.com/top200.htm.
3. Erin Finkelstein"National medical spending attributable to overweight and obesity: how much, and who's paying?" *Journal of Health Affair.* May 14, 2003; Oct. 20, 2004.

Chapter 2

1. Gallagher et al., "Healthy percentage body fat ranges: an approach for developing guidelines based on body mass index." *Americal Journal of Clinical Nutrition.* 2000; 72: 694–701.
2. Maltz, Maxwell. *Psycho-Cybernetics.* Mass Market Paperback. New York, NY, ©1989.

Chapter 3

1. Lacy, Brigitte. "Metabolism matters II—the mechanics of metabolism." PTontheNET. 1 April 2005.
2. http://www.lifetoolsforwomen.com/w/8-hormones.htm.

Chapter 4

1. Buemann, B., Toubro, S., and Astrup, A. "The effect of wine or beer versus a carbonated soft drink, served at a meal, on ad libitum energy intake." *International Journal of Obesity and Related Metabolic Disorders.* 2002; 26: 1367–1372.
2. Crovetti, R. "The influence of thermic effect of food on satiety." *American Journal of Clinical Nutrition.* July 1998; 52 (7): 482–8.
3. Couet, C., et al. "Effect of dietary fish oil on body fat mass and basal fat oxidation in healthy adults." *International Journal of Obesity.* 22 July 1997; 21: 637–643.

4. De Castro, J.M. "The time of day of food intake influences overall intake in humans." *Journal of Nutrition.* 2003; 134: 104–11.

5. Farshchi, H. "Deleterious effects of omitting breakfast on insulin sensitivity and fasting lipid profiles in healthy lean women." *American Journal of Clinical Nutrition.* February 2005; 81: 388–396.

6. Farshchi, H. Beneficial metabolic effects of regular meal frequency on dietary thermogenesis, insulin sensitivity, and fasting lipid profiles in healthy obese women." *American Journal of Clinical Nutrition.* January 2005; 81: 16–24.

7. Farshchi H.R., Taylor M.A., and Macdonald, I.A. "Regular meal frequency creates more appropriate insulin sensitivity and lipid profiles compared with irregular meal frequency in healthy lean women." *European Journal of Clinical Nutrition.* 2004; 58: 1071–7.

8. Flechtner-Mors, M., et al. "Effects of moderate consumption of white wine on weight loss in overweight and obese subjects." *International Journal of Obesity and Related Metabolic Disorders.* 2004; 28: 1420–1426.

9. Jenkins D.J.A., et al. "Nibbling versus gorging: metabolic advantages of increased meal frequency." *New England Journal of Medicine.* 1989; 321: 929–34.

10. Keim, N.L., et al. "Weight loss is greater with consumption of large morning meals and fat-free mass is preserved with large evening meals in women on a controlled weight reduction regimen." *Journal of Nutrition.* 1997; 127: 75–82.

11. Parks, E.J., and McCrory, M. "When to eat and how often." *American Journal of Clinical Nutrition.* January 2005; 81: 3–4.

12. Piers, L.S., et al. "Substitution of saturated with monounsaturated fat in a 4-week diet affects body weight and composition of overweight and obese men." *British Journal of Nutrition.* September 2003; 90(3): 717–27.

13. Siler, S.Q., Neese, R.A., and Hellerstein, M.K. "De novo lipogenesis, lipid kinetics, and whole-body lipid balances in humans after acute

alcohol consumption." *American Journal of Clinical Nutrition.* 1999; 70: 928–936.

14. Taubert, D. "Chocolate and Blood Pressure in Elderly Individuals With Isolated Systolic Hypertension." *The Journal of the American Medical Association.* August 27, 2003; 290: 1029–1030.
15. Serafini, M. "Nature." U.S. Department of Agriculture Nutrient Data Laboratory. August 28, 2003; 424: 1013.
16. Yunsheng, M. "Association between eating patterns and obesity in a free-living US adult population." *The American Journal of Epidemiology.* 2003; 158: 85–92.

Chapter 5

1. Dulloo A, et al. "Efficacy of a green tea extract rich in catechin polyphenols and caffeine in increasing 24-hour energy expenditure and fat oxidation in humans." *American Journal of Clinical Nutrition.* 1999. 70: 1040–45.

Chapter 6

1. Brand-Miller, J., Wolever T., Foster-Powell K., and Colagiuri, S. The New Glucose Revolution. New York: Marlowe & Company, 2003.
2. Bruce, S. and Crawford, B. *Cerealizing America: The unsweetened story of American breakfast cereals.* [city?] Faber & Faber, 1995.
3. McKeown, N.M., et al. "Whole-grain intake is favorably associated with metabolic risk factors for type 2 diabetes and cardiovascular disease in the Framingham Offspring Study." *American Journal of Clinical Nutrition.* August 2002; 76(2): 390–8.
4. Pauline Koh-Banerjee, et al. "Changes in whole-grain, bran, and cereal fiber consumption in relation to 8-y weight gain among men." *American Journal of Clinical Nutrition.* November 2004; 80: 1237–1245.
5. Wu, W et al. "Lipophilic and hydrophilic antioxidant capacities of common foods in the United States." *Journal of Agricultural Food Chemistry.* June 2004; 16:52(12): 4026–37.

6. Joanne L. Slavin, Jacobs, D., Marquart, L. and Wiemer, K. "The role of whole grains in disease prevention." *Journal of the American Dietetic Association.* July 2001; 101: 780–785.
7. Simin Liu, et al. "Relation between changes in intakes of dietary fiber and grain products and changes in weight and development of obesity among middle-aged women." *American Journal of Clinical Nutrition.* November 2003; 78: 920–927.

Chapter 7

1. Gannon, M.C., et al. "An increase in dietary protein improves the blood glucose response in persons with type 2 diabetes." *American Journal of Clinical Nutrition.* 2003; 78: 734–41.
2. http://lowcarbdiets.about.com/od/nutrition/a/protein.htm
3. http://www.bodyforlife2.com/incompleteprotein.htm.
4. http://www/hc-sc.gc.ca/fn-an/food-guide-aliment/index_e.html.

Chapter 8

1. Ross, L. et al. "Low-Fat Dietary Pattern and Risk of Invasive Breast Cancer: The Women's Health Initiative Randomized Controlled Dietary Modification Trial." *The Journal of the American Medical Association.* 2006; 295: 629–642.
2. Gardner, Christopher D. "Comparison of the Atkins, Zone, Ornish, and LEARN Diets for change in weight and related risk factors among overweight premenopausal women: the A to Z weight loss study: a randomized trial." *The Journal of the American Medical Association.* 2007; 297: 969–977.
3. Rozin, P. "The ecology of eating. Smaller portion sizes in France than in the United States help explain the French Paradox." *Psychological Science.* September, 2003; 14(5): 450.
4. Samaha, Frederick F., M.D. "A low-carbohydrate as compared with a low-fat diet in severe obesity." *The New England Journal of Medicine.*

May 22, 2003; 348(21): 2074–2081.

5. Piers, L.S., et al. "Substitution of saturated with monounsaturated fat in a 4-week diet affects body weight and composition of overweight and obese men." *British Journal of Nutrition.* September 2003; 90(3): 717–27.
6. Press release. "FDA announces qualified health claims for omega-3 fatty acids." U.S. Food and Drug Administration. September 8, 2004. Retrieved on July 10, 2006.
7. Gerster, H. "Can adults adequately convert alpha-linolenic acid (18: 3n-3) to eicosapentaenoic acid (20: 5n-3) and docosahexaenoic acid (22: 6n-3)?" *International Journal for Vitamin and Nutrition Research.* 1998; 68: 159–173.
8. http://www/whfoods.com/genpage.php?tname=foodspice&dbid=123.

Chapter 10

1. Couet et al. Effect on dietary fish oil on body fat mass and basal fat oxidation in healthy adults. *International Journal of Obesity.* 1997:21:637-43.
2. Gannon, M.C, et al. "An increase in dietary protein improves the blood glucose response in persons with type 2 diabetes." *American Journal of Nutrition.* 2003; 78: 734–41
3. Hill, A et al. "Combining fish-oil supplements with regular aerobic exercise improves body composition and cardiovascular disease risk factors." *American Journal of Clinical Nutrition.* Volume 85:1267-1274.
4. Rothman, R. "Patient understanding of food labels: the role of literacy and numeracy." *American Journal of Preventive Medicine.* November 2006; 31(5): 391–398.

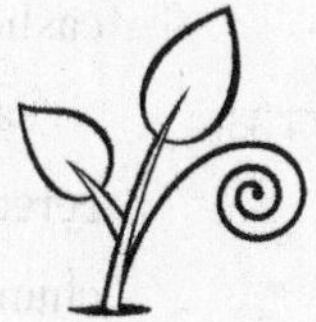

Index

A

B

C

G

H

I

J

K

L

M

N

O

P

Q

R

S

W

Y